N
P
F

Formulary

for Community Practitioners

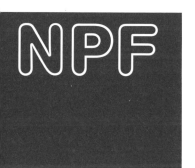

NPF

2009
2011

bnf.org

Published jointly by
BMJ Group
Tavistock Square, London WC1H 9JP, UK
and
RPS Publishing
RPS Publishing is the wholly-owned publishing organisation of the Royal Pharmaceutical Society of Great Britain
1 Lambeth High Street, London, SE1 7JN, UK

Copyright © BMJ Group and RPS Publishing 2009

ISBN: 978 0 85369 898 2

ISSN: 1468-4853

Printed by Pureprint Group, Uckfield, UK

Copies may be obtained through any bookseller or direct from:

Pharmaceutical Press
c/o Macmillan Distribution (MDL)
Brunel Rd
Houndmills
Basingstoke
RG21 6XS
UK
Tel: +44 (0) 1256 302 699
Fax: +44 (0) 1256 812 521
E-mail: direct@macmillan.co.uk
www.pharmpress.com

Contents

This edition of the NPF is intended as a pocket book for rapid reference and so cannot contain all the information necessary for patient management. For additional information the nurse prescriber should refer to the BNF or to the doctor who will have access to further information including manufacturers' product literature. Supplementary information is also available from pharmacists. Information can also be found in authoritative websites (follow links from http://bnf.org).

Preface

The Nurse Prescribers' Formulary for Community Practitioners (formerly the Nurse Prescribers' Formulary for District Nurses and Health Visitors) is for use by District Nurses and Specialist Community Public Health Nurses (including Health Visitors) who have received nurse prescriber training. It provides details of preparations that can be prescribed for patients receiving NHS treatment on form FP10P (form HS21(N) in Northern Ireland, form GP10(N) in Scotland, forms WP10CN and WP10PN in Wales).

Nurses who have received specific preparation and training (distinct from that provided to Community Practitioner nurse prescribers) and who are qualified as Nurse Independent Prescribers are able to prescribe any licensed medicine for any medical condition within their competence, including some Controlled Drugs. The current edition of the NPF includes a list of the Controlled Drugs and the indications for which they may be prescribed by Nurse Independent Prescribers. Further details may be found on the Department of Health website www.dh.gov.uk/nonmedicalprescribing

Community Practitioner nurse prescribers should prescribe only from the list of preparations in the Nurse Prescribers' Formulary for Community Practitioners (for conditions specified in the NPF). Most medicinal preparations should be prescribed by generic titles as shown under the individual monographs in the NPF; however, some medicinal preparations and a majority of appliances may need to be prescribed by brand name—see individual product entries in the NPF.

The Nurse Prescribers' Advisory Group (formerly the Nurse Prescribers' Formulary Subcommittee) (p. v) oversees the preparation of the NPF for Community Practitioners and advises the UK health ministers on the list of preparations that may be prescribed by Community Practitioner nurse prescribers.

The list of preparations from which Community Practitioner nurse prescribers may prescribe is reviewed constantly in the light of comments from nurse prescribers and applications from manufacturers.

The NPF has been designed for use with the British National Formulary (BNF); it forms an appendix to the BNF and as such is termed the Nurse Prescribers' Formulary Appendix (Appendix NPF). The current edition of the NPF includes Appendix 8 (Wound Management Products and Elasticated Garments) from BNF 58 (September 2009).

The Nurse Prescribers' Advisory Group records its thanks to BNF staff particularly E. Nix for their help with the preparation of this edition. J. E. Macintyre and staff provided valuable technical assistance. Xpage have provided assistance with typesetting.

The Subcommittee is grateful to those who have commented on previous editions of the NPF. In order that future editions of the NPF for Community Practitioners are able to reflect the requirements of nurse prescribers, users are urged to send comments and constructive criticism to:

NPF/BNF,
Royal Pharmaceutical Society of Great Britain
1 Lambeth High Street, London SE1 7JN.
editor@bnf.org

Nurses Prescribers' Advisory Group 2009

Chair

Nicky A. Cullum
PhD, RGN

Committee Members

Una J. Adderley
MSc, BA, RGN, DN

Rebecca F. Cheatle
BSc, RGN

Michele L. Cossey
BPharm, MSc, MRPharmS

Molly Courtenay
PhD, MSc, Cert Ed, BSc, RGN

Duncan S.T. Enright
MA, PGCE, MInstP, FIDM

Penny M. Franklin
RN, RCN, RSCPHN(HV), MA, PGCE

Margaret F. Helliwell
MB, BS, BSc, MFPHM FRCP (Edin)

Bryony Jordan
BSc, DipPharmPract, MRPharmS

Martin J. Kendall
OBE, MD, FRCP, FFPM

Fiona Lynch
BSc, MSc, RGN, RSCN

John Martin
BPharm, PhD, MRPharmS

Paul S. Maycock
MPharm, DipPharmPract, MRPharmS

Maureen P. Morgan
RN, RHV, MBA

Elizabeth J. Plastow
RMN, RGN, RSCPHN(HV), MSc, PGDipEd

Paul G. H. Robinson

Gul Root
BSc, MRPharmS, DMS

Jill M. Shearer
BSc, RGN, RM

Rabina Tindale
RGN, RSCN, BSc, DipAEN, PGCE

Vicky Vidler
MA, RGN, RSCN

Nurse Prescribers' Formulary for Community Practitioners

Prescription Writing

Further information may be found in BNF pp. 1–5

Prescriptions written by nurse prescribers should:

- be computer printed or written legibly in ink;
- be dated;
- state patient's full name and address;
- be signed in ink by the prescriber;
- include age and date of birth of patient.

Also recommended:

- Dose and the dose frequency should be stated. For preparations to be taken 'as required' **a minimum dose interval** should be specified, e.g. 'every 4 hours'.
- The unnecessary use of decimal points should be avoided, e.g. 3 mg, not 3.0 mg.
- Strength of the preparation should be stated, e.g. Paracetamol Tablets 500 mg.
- Quantities of 1 gram or more should be written as 1 g etc.
- Quantities of less than 1 gram should be written in milligrams, e.g. 500 mg, not 0.5 g (see inside back cover of BNF for conversion guide). It is, however, acceptable to express a range in the decimal form, e.g. 0.5 to 1 g.
- Quantity prescribed should generally be the pack size specified in the NPF under each preparation.
- Names of medicines should be written clearly using approved (generic) titles or proprietary names as specified throughout the NPF and should **not** be abbreviated.
- Directions should be in **English** and should not be abbreviated.

Security and validity of prescriptions

In order to ensure the security and validity of prescriptions nurse prescribers should:

- not leave them unattended;
- not leave them in a car where they may be visible;
- keep them locked up when not in use.

When there is any doubt about the authenticity of a prescription, the pharmacist will contact the nurse prescriber; see also Incomplete Prescriptions, below.

Children

Prescriptions should be written according to the guidelines above, stating the child's age.

Children's doses are stated in the NPF where appropriate but nurse prescribers should prescribe for children only if it is within their competence and after a full assessment (bearing in mind the differences in assessment between adults and children).

Where a single dose is stated for a given age range, it applies to the middle of the age range and may need to be adjusted to obtain doses for ages at the lower and upper limits of the stated range. Nurse prescribers are advised to err on the side of caution.

The pharmacist will supply an **oral syringe** with oral liquid preparations if the dose prescribed is less than 5 mL. The oral syringe is marked in 0.5-mL divisions from 1 to 5 mL to measure doses of less than 5 mL. It is provided with an adaptor and an instruction leaflet. A 5-mL spoon will be given for doses of 5 or 10 mL.

> For detailed advice on medicines for children consult *BNF for Children.*

Unlicensed and 'off-label' prescribing

In general the *doses, indications, cautions, contra-indications*, and *side-effects* in the NPF reflect those in the manufacturers' data sheets or Summaries of Product Characteristics (SPCs) which, in turn, reflect those in the corresponding marketing authorisations or product licences.

Community Practitioner Nurse Prescribers should not prescribe unlicensed medicines, that is, medicines without a valid marketing authorisation or product licence. Neither should they prescribe licensed medicines for uses, doses, or routes that are outside the product licence (unlicensed use, 'off-label' use, or 'off-licence' use). The only exception is nystatin which may be prescribed for neonates under certain circumstances (see p. 16).

Excipients

Where an oral liquid medicine in the NPF is available in a form free of *fructose, glucose,* or *sucrose* a note has been added to say that a sugar-free version may be requested by adding 'sugar free' to the prescription. Preparations containing hydrogenated glucose syrup, mannitol, maltitol, sorbitol, or xylitol are also marked 'sugar-free' because there is evidence that they do not cause dental caries. Whenever possible sugar-free preparations should be requested for children to reduce the risk of dental decay.

Where information on the presence of *aspartame, gluten, tartrazine, arachis (peanut) oil* or *sesame oil* is available, this is indicated against the relevant product entry; in the absence of information on excipients in the NPF or in the product literature, then the manufacturer should be contacted.

Information is provided on *selected excipients* in skin preparations (see BNF section 13.1.3).

Prevention of adverse reactions

Adverse reactions may be prevented as follows:

- Never prescribe any medicine unless there is a good indication.
- A Community Practitioner nurse prescriber should **not** prescribe medicines for pregnant women (except folic acid and, in some circumstances, nicotine replacement therapy); the patient should be referred to her doctor.
- It is very important to recognise allergy as a cause of adverse drug reactions. Ask if the patient has had any previous reactions, particularly when prescribing aspirin or dressings impregnated with iodine.
- Ask if the patient is taking any other medicines **including self medication**; remember that aspirin interacts with warfarin.
- Check whether there are any special instructions in relation to hepatic or renal disease.
- Prescribe as few medicines as possible and give very clear instructions to the elderly or any patient likely to misunderstand complicated instructions. Elderly patients cannot normally cope with more than three different medicines (and ideally they should not need to be taken more than twice daily).

Reporting of adverse reactions

If a patient has a suspected adverse reaction to a medicine or dressing, the nurse prescriber should consider reporting it to the Medicines and Healthcare products Regulatory Agency (MHRA) through the Yellow Card Scheme for reporting adverse reactions.

Yellow Cards for reporting are bound in this book (inside back cover); alternatively, an electronic form is available at www.yellowcard.gov.uk.

For more details on adverse reactions to drugs and on reporting, see BNF p.11.

Incomplete prescriptions

A pharmacist may need to contact the nurse prescriber if the *quantity*, *strength* or *dose* are missing from the prescription. The pharmacist will then arrange for the missing details to be added. Under some circumstances the pharmacist will use professional judgement as to what to give and will endorse the prescription.

Labelling of dispensed medicine

The following will appear on the label of a dispensed medicine:

- name of product
- name of patient
- date of dispensing
- name and address of pharmacy
- directions for use
- total quantity of product dispensed
- advice to keep out of reach of children.

Other information (e.g. 'flammable') will be added by the pharmacist as appropriate. Preparation entries in the NPF provide details of any additional cautionary advice that the pharmacist will add.

The *name of the product* will be that which is written on the prescription.

Safety in the home

Patients must be warned to keep all medicines out of the reach of children. Medicines will be dispensed in reclosable *child-resistant containers* unless:

- they are in manufacturers' original packs designed for supplying to the patient
- the patient would have difficulty in opening a child-resistant container.

In the latter case the pharmacist will make a particular point of advising that the medicines be kept out of reach of children. The nurse prescriber could usefully *reinforce this advice*.

Patients should be advised to dispose of *unwanted medicines* by returning them to a pharmacist for destruction.

Duplicate medicines

Nurses are well placed to check on whether patients are at risk of taking two medicines with the same action (or which contain the same ingredient) at the same time. This is of special concern in the case of medicines that can also be bought over the counter (e.g. aspirin and paracetamol). Pharmacists reduce this risk to some extent by making sure that the words 'aspirin' or 'aspirin and paracetamol' appear on relevant preparations. A check on the patient's medicines (including cough and cold preparations) might prevent the patient inadvertently taking duplicate doses of aspirin or paracetamol.

Prices

Net prices have been included in the NPF to provide an indication of relative cost. These prices are **not** suitable for quoting to patients since they do not include the pharmacist's professional fee and other allowances, nor do they include VAT.

PACT and SPA

PACT (Prescribing Analyses and Cost) and SPA (Scottish Prescribing Analysis) provide prescribers with information about their prescribing in comparison with the prescribing figures for the local Primary Care Trust equivalent practice and with a national equivalent. PACT is available electronically (www.nhsbsa.nhs.uk).

Changes to the Nurse Prescribers' List for Community Practitioners

Nurse Prescribers' Formulary

Additions

Medicinal preparations added to Nurse Prescribers' List since 2007

Doublebase® Emollient Bath Additive

Doublebase® Emollient Wash Gel

Gygel® Contraceptive Jelly

QV® Bath Oil

QV® Cream

QV® Lotion

QV® Wash

Deletions

Preparations deleted from the Nurse Prescribers' List since 2007

Alpha Keri® Bath Oil

Docusate Enema, Compound, BP

Decubal® Clinic

Keri® Therapeutic Lotion

Macrogol Oral Powder, NPF

Malathion alcoholic lotions containing at least 0.5%

Ortho-Crème® Cream

Phenothrin Alcoholic Lotion, NPF

Senna granules, Standardised, BP

Significant dose changes

Significant changes in dose statements introduced into NPF 2009–2011

Choline Salicylate Dental Gel, p. 17

Miconazole Oromucosal Gel, p. 16

> **Nurse Independent Prescribing**
> Nurses who have received specific training (distinct from that provided to Community Practitioner Nurse Prescribers) may prescribe any licensed medicine for any medical condition within their competence, including some Controlled Drugs, see p. 5.

Nurse Prescribers' Formulary for Community Practitioners

List of preparations approved by the Secretary of State which may be prescribed on form FP10P (form HS21(N) in Northern Ireland, form GP10(N) in Scotland, forms WP10CN and WP10PN in Wales) by Nurses for National Health Service patients.

Community Practitioners who have completed the necessary training may only prescribe items appearing in the nurse prescribers' list set out below. Community Practitioner Nurse Prescribers are recommended to prescribe generically, except where this would not be clinically appropriate or where there is no approved generic name.

Medicinal Preparations

Almond Oil Ear Drops, BP

Arachis Oil Enema, NPF

[1]Aspirin Tablets, Dispersible, 300 mg, BP

Bisacodyl Suppositories, BP (includes 5 mg and 10 mg strengths)

Bisacodyl Tablets, BP

Catheter Maintenance Solution, Chlorhexidine, NPF

Catheter Maintenance Solution, Sodium Chloride, NPF

Catheter Maintenance Solution, 'Solution G', NPF

Catheter Maintenance Solution, 'Solution R', NPF

Chlorhexidine Gluconate Alcoholic Solutions containing at least 0.05%

Chlorhexidine Gluconate Aqueous Solutions containing at least 0.05%

Choline Salicylate Dental Gel, BP

Clotrimazole Cream 1%, BP

Co-danthramer Capsules, NPF

Co-danthramer Capsules, Strong, NPF

Co-danthramer Oral Suspension, NPF

Co-danthramer Oral Suspension, Strong, NPF

Co-danthrusate Capsules, BP

Co-danthrusate Oral Suspension, NPF

Crotamiton Cream, BP

Crotamiton Lotion, BP

Dimeticone barrier creams containing at least 10%

Dimeticone Lotion, NPF

Docusate Capsules, BP

Docusate Enema, NPF

Docusate Oral Solution, BP

Docusate Oral Solution, Paediatric, BP

Econazole Cream 1%, BP

Emollients as listed below:

    Aqueous Cream, BP

    Arachis Oil, BP

    Cetraben® Emollient Cream

    Dermamist®

    Diprobase® Cream

    Diprobase® Ointment

    Doublebase®

    E45® Cream

    Emulsifying Ointment, BP

---

1. Max. 96 tablets; max. pack size 32 tablets

Hydromol® Cream
Hydromol® Ointment
Hydrous Ointment, BP
Linola® Gamma Cream
Lipobase®
Liquid and White Soft Paraffin Ointment, NPF
Neutrogena® Norwegian Formula Dermatological
 Cream
Oilatum® Cream
Oilatum® Junior Cream
Paraffin, White Soft, BP
Paraffin, Yellow Soft, BP
QV® Cream
QV® Lotion
QV® Wash
Ultrabase®
Unguentum M®
Zerobase® Cream
Emollient Bath Additives as listed below:
 [1]Balneum®
 Cetraben® Emollient Bath Additive
 Dermalo® Bath Emollient
 Diprobath®
 Doublebase® Emollient Bath Additive
 Doublebase® Emollient Shower Gel
 Doublebase® Emollient Wash Gel
 Hydromol® Bath and Shower Emollient
 Imuderm® Bath Oil
 Oilatum® Emollient
 Oilatum® Junior Emollient Bath Additive
 Oilatum® Gel
 QV® Bath Oil
Folic Acid 400 micrograms/5 mL Oral Solution, NPF
Folic Acid Tablets 400 micrograms, BP
Glycerol Suppositories, BP
[2]Ibuprofen Oral Suspension, BP
[2]Ibuprofen Tablets, BP
Ispaghula Husk Granules, BP
Ispaghula Husk Granules, Effervescent, BP
Ispaghula Husk Oral Powder, BP
Lactulose Solution, BP
Lidocaine Ointment, BP
Lidocaine and Chlorhexidine Gel, BP
Macrogol Oral Powder, Compound, NPF
Macrogol Oral Powder, Compound, Half-strength, NPF
Magnesium Hydroxide Mixture, BP
Magnesium Sulphate Paste, BP
Malathion aqueous lotions containing at least 0.5%
Mebendazole Oral Suspension, NPF
Mebendazole Tablets, NPF
Methylcellulose Tablets, BP
Miconazole Cream 2%, BP
Miconazole Oromucosal Gel, BP
Mouthwash Solution-tablets, NPF
Nicotine Inhalation Cartridge for Oromucosal Use, NPF
Nicotine Lozenge, NPF
Nicotine Medicated Chewing Gum, NPF
Nicotine Nasal Spray, NPF
Nicotine Sublingual Tablets, NPF
Nicotine Transdermal Patches, NPF
Nystatin Oral Suspension, BP
Olive Oil Ear Drops, BP
Paracetamol Oral Suspension, BP (includes 120 mg/
 5 mL and 250 mg/5 mL strengths—both of which are
 available as sugar-free formulations)

[3]Paracetamol Tablets, BP
[3]Paracetamol Tablets, Soluble, BP (includes 120-mg and
 500-mg tablets)
Permethrin Cream, NPF
Phenothrin Aqueous Lotion, NPF
Phosphate Suppositories, NPF
Phosphates Enema, BP
Piperazine and Senna Powder, NPF
Povidone–Iodine Solution, BP
Senna Oral Solution, NPF
Senna Tablets, BP
Senna and Ispaghula Granules, NPF
Sodium Chloride Solution, Sterile, BP
Sodium Citrate Compound Enema, NPF
Sodium Picosulfate Capsules, NPF
Sodium Picosulfate Elixir, NPF
Spermicidal contraceptives as listed below:
 Gygel® Contraceptive Jelly
Sterculia Granules, NPF
Sterculia and Frangula Granules, NPF
Titanium Ointment, BP
Water for Injections, BP
Zinc and Castor Oil Ointment, BP
Zinc Cream, BP
Zinc Ointment, BP
Zinc Oxide and Dimeticone Spray, NPF
Zinc Oxide Impregnated Medicated Bandage, NPF
Zinc Oxide Impregnated Medicated Stocking, NPF
Zinc Paste Bandage, BP 1993
Zinc Paste and Calamine Bandage
Zinc Paste and Ichthammol Bandage, BP 1993

Appliances and Reagents (including Wound Management Products)

Community Practitioner Nurse Prescribers in England, Wales and Northern Ireland can prescribe any appliance or reagent in the relevant Drug Tariff. In the Scottish Drug Tariff, Appliances and Reagents which may **not** be prescribed by Nurses are annotated **Nx**.

Appliances (including Contraceptive Devices[4]) as listed in Part IXA of the Drug Tariff (Part III of the Northern Ireland Drug Tariff, Part 3 (Appliances) and Part 2 (Dressings) of the Scottish Drug Tariff)

Incontinence Appliances as listed in Part IXB of the Drug Tariff (Part III of the Northern Ireland Drug Tariff, Part 5 of the Scottish Drug Tariff)

Stoma Appliances and Associated Products as listed in Part IXC of the Drug Tariff (Part III of the Northern Ireland Drug Tariff, Part 6 of the Scottish Drug Tariff)

Chemical Reagents as listed in Part IXR of the Drug Tariff (Part II of the Northern Ireland Drug Tariff, Part 9 of the Scottish Drug Tariff)

The Drug Tariffs can be accessed online at:
National Health Service Drug Tariff for England and Wales: www.ppa.org.uk/ppa/edt_intro.htm
Health and Personal Social Services for Northern Ireland Drug Tariff: www.centralservicesagency.com/display/ni_drug_tariff
Scottish Drug Tariff: www.isdscotland.org/isd/2245.html

---

1. Except pack sizes that are not to be prescribed under the NHS (see Part XVIIIA of the Drug Tariff, Part XI of the Northern Ireland Drug Tariff)
2. Except for indications and doses that are PoM

3. Max. 96 tablets; max. pack size 32 tablets
4. Nurse Prescribers in Family Planning Clinics—where it is not appropriate for nurse prescribers in family planning clinics to prescribe contraceptive devices using form FP10P (forms WP10CN and WP10PN in Wales), they may prescribe using the same system as doctors in the clinic

Nurse Independent Prescribing

Nurse Independent Prescribers (formerly known as Extended Formulary Nurse Prescribers) are able to prescribe any licensed medicine for any medical condition, including some Controlled Drugs (see below).

Nurse Independent Prescribers must work within their own level of professional competence and expertise. They are recommended to prescribe generically, except where this would not be clinically appropriate or where there is no approved non-proprietary name.

Nurse Independent Prescribers are also able to prescribe independently the Controlled Drugs in the table below, *solely for the medical conditions indicated.*

Up-to-date information and guidance on nurse independent prescribing is available on the Department of Health website at www.dh.gov.uk/nonmedicalprescribing

Controlled drugs prescribable by Nurse Independent Prescribers solely for the medical conditions indicated

Drug	Indication	Route of Administration
Buprenorphine	Transdermal use in palliative care	Transdermal
Chlordiazepoxide hydrochloride	Treatment of initial or acute withdrawal symptoms caused by the withdrawal of alcohol from persons habituated to it	Oral
Codeine phosphate	–	Oral
Co-phenotrope	–	Oral
Diamorphine hydrochloride	Use in palliative care, pain relief in respect of suspected myocardial infarction or for relief of acute or severe pain after trauma, including in either case postoperative pain relief	Oral, parenteral
Diazepam	Use in palliative care, treatment of initial or acute withdrawal symptoms caused by the withdrawal of alcohol from persons habituated to it, tonic-clonic seizures	Oral, parenteral, rectal
Dihydrocodeine tartrate	–	Oral
Fentanyl	Transdermal use in palliative care	Transdermal
Lorazepam	Use in palliative care, tonic-clonic seizures	Oral, parenteral
Midazolam	Use in palliative care, tonic-clonic seizures	Parenteral, buccal
Morphine hydrochloride	Use in palliative care, pain relief in respect of suspected myocardial infarction or for relief of acute or severe pain after trauma, including in either case postoperative pain relief	Rectal
Morphine sulphate	Use in palliative care, pain relief in respect of suspected myocardial infarction or for relief of acute or severe pain after trauma, including in either case postoperative pain relief	Oral, parenteral, rectal
Oxycodone hydrochloride	Use in palliative care	Oral, parenteral

Note For the purposes of nurse independent prescribing, palliative care means the care of patients with advanced, progressive illness

Laxatives

Corresponds to BNF section 1.6.

Before prescribing laxatives it is important to be sure that the patient *is* constipated and that the constipation is *not* secondary to an underlying undiagnosed complaint.

It is also important for those who complain of constipation to understand that bowel habit can vary considerably in frequency without doing harm. Some people may consider themselves constipated if they do not have a bowel movement each day. A useful definition of constipation is the passage of hard stools less frequently than the patient's own normal pattern and this can be explained to the patient.

Misconceptions about bowel habits have led to excessive laxative use. Abuse may lead to hypokalaemia. *Simple constipation* is usually relieved by increasing the intake of dietary fibre and fluids.

Laxatives should generally be **avoided** except where straining will exacerbate a condition (such as angina) or increase the risk of rectal bleeding as in haemorrhoids. Laxatives are also of value in *drug-induced constipation*, for the *expulsion of parasites* after anthelmintic treatment, and to clear the alimentary tract *before surgery and radiological procedures*. Prolonged treatment of constipation is sometimes necessary.

Children Laxatives should be prescribed by a healthcare professional experienced in the management of constipation in children. Delays of greater than 3 days between stools may increase the likelihood of pain on passing hard stools leading to anal fissure, anal spasm and eventually to a learned response to avoid defaecation. Increased fluid and fibre intake may be sufficient to regulate bowel action.

> Community Practitioner nurse prescribers should discuss with the doctor before prescribing a laxative for a child

Laxatives can be divided into four main groups: *bulk-forming laxatives*, *stimulant laxatives*, *faecal softeners*, and *osmotic laxatives*. This simple classification, however, disguises the fact that some laxatives have complex actions.

Bulk-forming laxatives

Bulk-forming laxatives relieve constipation by increasing faecal mass which stimulates peristalsis. Patients should be told that the full effect may take some days to develop. In nursing practice they are particularly useful in the management of patients with *colostomy, ileostomy, haemorrhoids*, and *anal fissure*. Methylcellulose tablets are licensed for other indications including diarrhoea and obesity but nurse prescribers should prescribe them **only** for constipation.

BULK-FORMING LAXATIVES

Indications constipation, see also notes above

Cautions adequate fluid intake should be maintained to avoid intestinal obstruction—it may be necessary to supervise elderly or debilitated patients or those with intestinal narrowing or decreased motility

Contra-indications difficulty in swallowing, intestinal obstruction, colonic atony, faecal impaction; avoid methylcellulose in infective bowel disease

Side-effects flatulence, abdominal distension; gastro-intestinal obstruction or impaction; hypersensitivity reported

Dose
- See preparations, below

> **Counselling**
> Preparations that swell in contact with liquid should always be carefully swallowed with water and should not be taken immediately before going to bed

◢*Prescribe as:*

Ispaghula Husk Granules (*Fibrelief*)

Granules, sugar- and gluten-free, ispaghula husk 3.5 g/sachet (natural or orange flavour), net price 10 sachets = £1.23, 30 sachets = £2.07.
Excipients include aspartame (see BNF section 9.4.1)
Dose ADULT and CHILD over 12 years, 1–6 sachets daily in water in 1–3 divided doses

Ispaghula Husk Granules (*Isogel*)

Granules, brown, sugar- and gluten-free, ispaghula husk 90%, net price 200 g = £2.67.
Dose 2 level 5-mL spoonfuls in water once or twice daily, preferably at mealtimes; CHILD (but see notes above) 1 level 5-mL spoonful in water once or twice daily, preferably at meal times
Note May be difficult to obtain

Ispaghula Husk Oral Powder (*Regulan*)

Powder, beige, sugar- and gluten-free, ispaghula husk 3.4 g/5.85-g sachet (orange or lemon/lime flavour), net price 30 sachets = £2.44.
Excipients include aspartame (see BNF section 9.4.1)
Dose 1 sachet in 150 mL water 1–3 times daily; CHILD (but see notes above) 6–12 years 2.5–5 mL in water 1–3 times daily

Effervescent Ispaghula Husk Granules (*Fybogel*)

Granules, buff, effervescent, sugar- and gluten-free, ispaghula husk 3.5 g/sachet, net price 30 sachets (lemon or orange flavour or plain) = £1.84
Excipients include aspartame 16 mg/sachet (see BNF section 9.4.1)
Dose 1 sachet or 2 level 5-mL spoonfuls in water twice daily, preferably after meals; CHILD (but see notes above) 6–12 years ½–1 level 5 mL spoonful in water, twice daily

Effervescent Ispaghula Husk Granules (*Ispagel Orange*)

Granules, beige, effervescent, sugar- and gluten-free, ispaghula husk 3.5 g/sachet (orange flavour), net price 30 sachets = £2.10.
Excipients include aspartame (see BNF section 9.4.1)
Dose 1 sachet in water 1–3 times daily; CHILD (but see notes above) 6–12 years half adult dose

Methylcellulose Tablets

Tablets, pink, scored, methylcellulose '450' 500 mg, net price 112-tab pack = £3.22. *Proprietary product: Celevac tablets*
Dose 3–6 tablets twice daily with at least 300 mL of liquid

Sterculia Granules

Granules, coated, gluten-free, sterculia 62%, net price 500 g = £5.94; 60 × 7-g sachets = £4.99. *Proprietary product: Normacol*

Dose 1–2 heaped 5-mL spoonfuls or contents of 1–2 sachets, washed down without chewing with plenty of liquid once or twice daily after meals; CHILD (but see notes above) 6–12 years half adult dose

Sterculia and Frangula Granules

Granules, brown, coated, gluten-free, sterculia 62%, frangula (standardised) 8%, net price 500 g = £6.34; 60 × 7-g sachets = £5.34. *Proprietary product: Normacol Plus*

Dose 1–2 heaped 5-mL spoonfuls or contents of 1–2 sachets, washed down without chewing with plenty of liquid once or twice daily after meals

---

Stimulant laxatives

Stimulant laxatives increase intestinal motility and are used in functional constipation that has not responded to dietary measures.

Stimulant laxatives often cause abdominal cramp. They should be avoided in intestinal obstruction, and prolonged use can cause diarrhoea and related effects such as hypokalaemia. They should preferably be avoided in children.

> Community Practitioner nurse prescribers should discuss with the doctor before prescribing a laxative for a child

> Cross-references to the BNF are provided but nurse prescribers may only prescribe those items that are listed on the Nurse Prescribers' list.

▋ BISACODYL

Indications constipation; tablets act in 10–12 hours; suppositories act in 20–60 minutes

Cautions see notes on stimulant laxatives

Contra-indications see notes on stimulant laxatives; acute surgical abdominal conditions, acute inflammatory bowel disease, severe dehydration

Side-effects see notes on stimulant laxatives; nausea and vomiting; colitis also reported; *suppositories*, local irritation

Dose

- See under preparations, below

◀*Prescribe as:*

Bisacodyl Tablets 5 mg

Tablets, enteric coated, bisacodyl 5 mg. Net price 100 = £3.27

Dose 1–2 tablets at night; CHILD (but see notes above) 4–10 years (on doctor's advice only) 1 tablet at night, over 10 years 1–2 tablets at night

Bisacodyl Suppositories 10 mg

Suppositories, bisacodyl 10 mg. Net price 12 = 89p

Dose 1 suppository rectally in the morning, CHILD over 10 years (but see notes above) 1 suppository rectally in the morning

Bisacodyl Paediatric Suppositories 5 mg

Paediatric suppositories, bisacodyl 5 mg. Net price 5 = 94p

Dose CHILD (but see notes above) under 10 years 1 suppository rectally in the morning (on doctor's advice only)

▋ DANTRON

(Danthron)

Indications in consultation with doctor, only for: constipation in terminally ill patients of all ages; acts within 6–12 hours

Cautions see notes on stimulant laxatives; avoid prolonged contact with skin (as in incontinent patients)—risk of irritation and excoriation; *rodent* studies indicate potential carcinogenic risk

Contra-indications see notes on stimulant laxatives; pregnancy (BNF Appendix 4); breast-feeding (BNF Appendix 5)

Side-effects see notes on stimulant laxatives; urine may be coloured red

Dose

- See under preparations

◀*Prescribe as:*

Co-danthramer Capsules [PoM]

Capsules, co-danthramer 25/200 (dantron 25 mg, poloxamer '188' 200 mg). Net price 60-cap pack = £12.86

Dose (restricted indications, see above) 1–2 capsules at bedtime; CHILD 1 capsule at bedtime

Strong Co-danthramer Capsules [PoM]

Capsules, co-danthramer 37.5/500 (dantron 37.5 mg, poloxamer '188' 500 mg). Net price 60-cap pack = £15.55

Dose (restricted indications, see above) 1–2 capsules at bedtime; CHILD under 12 years not recommended

Co-danthramer Oral Suspension [PoM]

Oral suspension, co-danthramer 25/200 in 5 mL (dantron 25 mg, poloxamer '188' 200 mg/5 mL). Net price 300 mL = £11.27, 1 litre = £37.57

Dose (restricted indications, see above) 5–10 mL at night; CHILD 2.5–5 mL

Strong Co-danthramer Oral Suspension [PoM]

Strong oral suspension, co-danthramer 75/1000 in 5 mL (dantron 75 mg, poloxamer '188' 1 g/5 mL). Net price 300 mL = £30.13

Dose (restricted indications, see above) 5 mL at night; CHILD under 12 years not recommended

Co-danthrusate Capsules [PoM]

Capsules, co-danthrusate 50/60 (dantron 50 mg, docusate sodium 60 mg). Net price 63-cap pack = £14.50

Dose (restricted indications, see above) 1–3 capsules, usually at night; CHILD 6–12 years 1 capsule at night

Co-danthrusate Oral Suspension [PoM]

Oral suspension, yellow, co-danthrusate 50/60 in 5 mL (dantron 50 mg, docusate sodium 60 mg/5 mL). Net price 200 mL = £8.75.

Dose (restricted indications, see above) 5–15 mL at night; CHILD 6–12 years 5 mL at night

DOCUSATE SODIUM
(Dioctyl Sodium Sulphosuccinate)

Indications   constipation (oral preparations act within 1–2 days)

Cautions   see notes on stimulant laxatives; do not give with liquid paraffin; rectal preparations not indicated if haemorrhoids or anal fissure; pregnancy (BNF Appendix 4); breast-feeding (BNF Appendix 5)

Contra-indications   see notes on stimulant laxatives

Side-effects   see notes on stimulant laxatives

Dose

- see under preparations
  Note Docusate preparations probably also have faecal softening effect.

◀*Prescribe as:*
Docusate Capsules 100 mg
Capsules, yellow/white, docusate sodium 100 mg, net price 30-cap pack = £1.92, 100-cap pack = £6.40. *Proprietary product: Dioctyl Capsules*
Dose up to 5 capsules daily in divided doses

Docusate Oral Solution 50 mg/5 mL
Oral solution, sugar-free, docusate sodium 50 mg/5 mL. Net price 300-mL = £5.49. *Proprietary product: Docusol Adult Solution*
Dose up to 50 mL daily in divided doses

Paediatric Docusate Oral Solution 12.5 mg/5 mL
Paediatric oral solution, sugar-free, docusate sodium 12.5 mg/5 mL. Net price 300 mL = £5.29. *Proprietary product: Docusol Paediatric Solution*
Dose CHILD (but see notes above) 6 months–2 years 5 mL 3 times daily, 2–12 years 5–10 mL 3 times daily

Docusate Enema
Enema, docusate sodium 120 mg in 10-g single-dose disposable packs. Net price 10-g unit = 57p. *Proprietary product: Norgalax Micro-enema*
Dose ADULT and CHILD (but see notes above) over 12 years, 10-g unit

GLYCEROL
(Glycerin)

Indications   constipation

Dose

- See under preparations

◀*Prescribe as:*
Glycerol Suppositories
(Synonym: Glycerin Suppositories)
Suppositories, gelatin 140 mg, glycerol (glycerin) 700 mg/g. Net price 12 × 1-g = £1.04; 12 × 2-g = £1.02; 12 × 4-g = £1.47
Dose 1 suppository moistened with water before use, when required
The usual sizes are INFANT under 1 year, small (1-g mould), CHILD 1–12 years medium (2-g mould), ADULT and CHILD over 12 years, large (4-g mould)

SENNA

Indications   constipation (acts within 8–12 hours)

Cautions   see notes on stimulant laxatives

Contra-indications   see notes on stimulant laxatives

Side-effects   see notes on stimulant laxatives

Dose

- See under preparations

◀*Prescribe as:*
Senna Tablets
Tablets, total sennosides (calculated as sennoside B) 7.5 mg. Net price 60 = £1.89
Dose 2–4 tablets, usually at bedtime; initial dose should be low and then gradually increased; CHILD (but see notes above) 6–12 years, half adult dose in the morning (on doctor's advice only)
Note For senna tablets on general sale to the public lower dose recommended

Senna Oral Solution
Syrup, brown, total sennosides (calculated as sennoside B) 7.5 mg/5 mL. Net price 500 mL = £2.69 *Proprietary product: Senokot Syrup*
Dose 10–20 mL, usually at bedtime; CHILD (but see notes above) 2–6 years 2.5–5 mL in the morning (on doctor's advice only), 6–12 years, 5–10 mL in the morning
Note For senna oral solution on general sale to the public lower dose recommended

Senna and Ispaghula Granules
Granules, coated, senna fruit 12.4%, ispaghula 54.2%. Contain ispaghula as a bulk laxative. Net price 400 g = £7.45. *Proprietary product: Manevac Granules*
Dose 1–2 level 5-mL spoonfuls with water *or* warm drink after supper and, if necessary, before breakfast *or* every 6 hours in resistant cases for 1–3 days; CHILD (but see notes above) 5–12 years 1 level 5-mL spoonful daily
Counselling Preparations that swell in contact with liquid should always be carefully swallowed with water and should not be taken immediately before going to bed

SODIUM PICOSULFATE
(Sodium Picosulphate)

Indications   constipation (acts within 6–12 hours)

Cautions   see notes on stimulant laxatives; active inflammatory bowel disease (avoid if fulminant); breast-feeding (see BNF Appendix 5)

Contra-indications   see notes on stimulant laxatives; severe dehydration

Side-effects   see notes on stimulant laxatives

Dose

- See under preparations

◀*Prescribe as:*
Sodium Picosulfate Capsules
Capsules, sodium picosulfate 2.5 mg, net price 20-cap pack = £1.93, 50-cap pack = £2.73. *Proprietary product:* [1]*Dulcolax Perles*
Dose 2–4 capsules at night; CHILD (but see notes above) 4–10 years 1–2 capsules at night (on doctor's advice only), over 10 years 2–4 capsules at night

1. The brand name Dulcolax® is also used for bisacodyl tablets and suppositories

Sodium Picosulfate Elixir

Elixir, sodium picosulfate 5 mg/5 mL. Net price 100 mL = £1.85. *Proprietary product*: [1]*Dulcolax Liquid*

Dose 5–10 mL at night; CHILD (but see notes above), under 4 years 250 micrograms/kg (max. 5 mg) at night (on doctor's advice only), 4–10 years 2.5–5 mL at night (on doctor's advice only), over 10 years 5–10 mL at night

1. The brand name Dulcolax® is also used for bisacodyl tablets and suppositories

Faecal softeners

Faecal softeners, such as enemas containing arachis oil (ground-nut oil, peanut oil), lubricate and soften impacted faeces and promote a bowel movement.

 ARACHIS OIL

Indications constipation, see also notes above
Dose
- See under preparation

◢*Prescribe as:*
Arachis Oil Enema

Enema, arachis (peanut) oil in 130-mL single-dose disposable packs. Net price 130 mL = £7.98

Dose to soften impacted faeces, 130 mL; the enema should be warmed before use; CHILD on doctor's advice only

Osmotic laxatives

Osmotic laxatives increase the amount of water in the large bowel, either by drawing fluid from the body into the bowel or by retaining the fluid they were administered with.

Lactulose is a semi-synthetic disaccharide which is not absorbed from the gastro-intestinal tract. It is contra-indicated in galactosaemia and in intestinal obstruction; side-effects include flatulence, abdominal cramps and discomfort.

Macrogol (polyethylene glycol) may be used by mouth for constipation and the short-term treatment of faecal impaction. It is important that the initial assessment of faecal impaction is undertaken by a doctor. Macrogols sequester fluid in the bowel; giving fluid with macrogols may reduce the dehydrating effect sometimes seen with osmotic laxatives.

Magnesium hydroxide mixture is suitable for occasional use provided an adequate fluid intake is maintained after it has been given. It may be used when a rapid action is required but should be prescribed with caution because it is often abused.

Phosphate enemas are useful in bowel clearance before radiology, endoscopy, and surgery.

> Community Practitioner nurse prescribers should discuss with the doctor before prescribing a laxative for a child

 LACTULOSE

Indications constipation (may take up to 48 hours to act)
Cautions lactose intolerance; **interactions:** BNF Appendix 1 (lactulose)
Contra-indications galactosaemia, intestinal obstruction
Side-effects flatulence, cramps, and abdominal discomfort
Dose
- See under preparation

◢*Prescribe as:*
Lactulose Solution

Solution, lactulose 3.1–3.7 g/5 mL with other ketoses. Net price 300-mL pack = £2.64, 500-mL pack = £2.95

Dose initially 15 mL twice daily, adjusted according to patient's needs; CHILD (but see notes above) under 1 year 2.5 mL twice daily, 1–5 years 5 mL twice daily, 5–10 years 10 mL twice daily

 MACROGOLS
(Polyethylene glycols)

Indications constipation; faecal impaction (**only after** initial assessment by medical practitioner)
Cautions pregnancy and breast-feeding (see BNF Appendixes 4 and 5); discontinue if symptoms of fluid and electrolyte disturbance, see also preparations below
Contra-indications intestinal perforation or obstruction, paralytic ileus, severe inflammatory conditions of the intestinal tract (such as Crohn's disease, ulcerative colitis, and toxic megacolon)
Side-effects abdominal distension and pain, nausea
Dose
- See under preparations

◢*Prescribe as:*
Compound Macrogol Oral Powder

Oral powder, macrogol '3350' (polyethylene glycol '3350') 13.125 g, sodium bicarbonate 178.5 mg, sodium chloride 350.7 mg, potassium chloride 46.6 mg/sachet, net price 20-sachet pack (lime- and lemon-, or orange-, or plain-flavoured) = £4.45, 30-sachet pack (lime- and lemon-, or orange-, or chocolate-, or plain-flavoured) = £6.68, 50-sachet pack (lime- and lemon-, or plain-flavoured) = £11.13. *Proprietary products: Movicol, Laxido*

Note Amount of potassium chloride varies according to flavour of *Movicol®* as follows: plain-flavour (sugar-free) = 50.2 mg/sachet; lime and lemon flavour = 46.6 mg/sachet; chocolate flavour = 31.7 mg/sachet. 1 sachet when reconstituted with 125 mL water provides K⁺ 5.4 mmol/litre

Not to be confused with a preparation also containing sodium sulphate which is used for bowel cleansing before surgery and bowel procedures

Cautions patients with cardiovascular impairment should not take more than 2 sachets in any 1 hour

Dose chronic constipation, 1–3 sachets daily in divided doses usually for up to 2 weeks; contents of each sachet dissolved in half a glass (approx. 125 mL) of water; maintenance, 1–2 sachets daily; CHILD under 12 years not recommended

Faecal impaction (**important**: initial assessment by doctor), 8 sachets daily dissolved in 1 litre of water; the solution should be drunk within 6 hours, usually for max. 3 days; CHILD under 12 years not recommended

After reconstitution the solution should be kept in a refrigerator and discarded if unused after 6 hours

Compound Macrogol Oral Powder, Half-Strength

Oral powder, macrogol '3350' (polyethylene glycol '3350') 6.563 g, sodium bicarbonate 89.3 mg, sodium chloride 175.4 mg, potassium chloride 23.3 mg/sachet, net price 20-sachet pack (lime and lemon flavour) = £2.67, 30-sachet pack = £4.01. *Proprietary product: Movicol-Half*

Note *Movicol Paediatric Plain* is PoM and is **not** on the NPF list

Cautions patients with cardiovascular impairment should not take more than 4 sachets in any 1 hour

Dose chronic constipation, 2–6 sachets daily in divided doses usually for up to 2 weeks; content of each sachet dissolved in quarter of a glass (approx. 60–65 mL) water; maintenance, 2–4 sachets daily; CHILD under 12 years not recommended

Faecal impaction (**important**: initial assessment by doctor), 16 sachets daily dissolved in 1 litre of water and drunk within 6 hours, usually for max. 3 days; CHILD under 12 years not recommended. After reconstitution the solution should be kept in a refrigerator and discarded if unused after 6 hours

◼ MAGNESIUM HYDROXIDE

Indications constipation

Cautions renal impairment (see BNF Appendix 3; risk of magnesium accumulation); hepatic impairment (see BNF Appendix 2); elderly and debilitated; see also notes above; **interactions**: see BNF Appendix 1 (antacids)

Contra-indications acute gastro-intestinal conditions

Side-effects colic

Dose

• See under preparation

◀*Prescribe as:*

Magnesium Hydroxide Mixture

(Synonym: Cream of Magnesia)

Mixture, aqueous suspension containing about 8% of hydrated magnesium oxide. Do not store in a cold place

Dose constipation, ADULT and CHILD over 12 years, 30–45 mL with water at bedtime when required; CHILD (but see notes above) 3–12 years, 5–10 mL with water at bedtime when required

◼ PHOSPHATES (RECTAL)

Indications rectal use in constipation, see also notes above

Cautions see notes above; also elderly and debilitated; *with enema*, electrolyte disturbances, renal impairment, congestive heart failure, ascites, uncontrolled hypertension, maintain adequate hydration

Contra-indications acute gastro-intestinal conditions (including gastro-intestinal obstruction, inflammatory bowel disease, and conditions associated with increased colonic absorption)

Side-effects local irritation; *with enema*, electrolyte disturbances

Dose

• See under preparations

◀*Prescribe as:*

Phosphate Suppositories

Suppositories, sodium acid phosphate (anhydrous) 1.3 g, sodium bicarbonate 1.08 g, net price 12 = £2.01. *Proprietary product: Carbalax*

Dose constipation, 1 suppository, inserted 30 minutes before evacuation required; moisten with water before use; CHILD under 12 years not recommended

Phosphates Enema (Formula B)

Enema, sodium dihydrogen phosphate dihydrate 12.8 g, disodium phosphate dodecahydrate 10.24 g/128 mL. Net price 128 mL with standard tube = £2.98, with long rectal tube = £3.98

Dose 128 mL; CHILD (but see notes above) over 3 years, reduced according to body weight (under 3 years not recommended)

Phosphates Enema (*Fleet*)

Enema, sodium acid phosphate 21.4 g, sodium phosphate 9.4 g/118 mL. Net price single-dose pack (standard tube) = 46p

Dose ADULT and CHILD over 12 years, 118 mL; CHILD (but see notes above) 3–12 years, on doctor's advice only (under 3 years not recommended)

◼ SODIUM CITRATE (RECTAL)

Indications rectal use in constipation

Cautions elderly and debilitated; see also notes above

Contra-indications acute gastro-intestinal conditions

Dose

• See under preparations

◀*Prescribe as:*

Sodium Citrate Compound Enema

Enema, sodium citrate 450 mg with other ingredients including glycerol, sorbitol and an anionic surfactant in a 5-mL single-dose disposable pack. *Proprietary products: Micolette Micro-enema* (net price 5-mL pack = 38p), *Micralax Micro-enema* (5-mL pack = 41p), *Relaxit Micro-enema* (5-mL pack = 32p)

Dose ADULT and CHILD (but see notes above) over 3 years, 5 mL (under 3 years not recommended)

Gloves

◼ GLOVES

EMA Film Gloves, Disposable

Gloves, small, medium, or large. Net price pack of 30 = £2.40, pack of 100 = £3.27. *Proprietary product: Dispos-A-Gloves*

For use as a barrier during manual evacuation of the bowel

Nitrile Gloves

Gloves, extra small, small, medium, large, or extra large, net price pack of 50 = £3.89, 100 = £4.50

Polythene Gloves

Gloves, net price pack of 25 = 55p.

For use as occlusives with medicated creams

Analgesics

Corresponds to BNF section 4.7.1 (non-opioid analgesics) and 10.1.1 (non-steroidal anti-inflammatory drugs)

The **non-opioid** analgesics **aspirin**, **ibuprofen** and **paracetamol** are particularly suitable for pain in musculoskeletal conditions, whereas the opioid analgesics are more suitable for moderate to severe visceral pain. Aspirin, ibuprofen, and paracetamol are effective analgesics for the relief of *mild to moderate pain*. Their familiar role as household remedies should not detract from their considerable value as analgesics; they are also of value in some forms of *severe chronic pain*.

Combinations of aspirin or paracetamol with an opioid analgesic (such as codeine) are commonly used but their advantages have not been substantiated (and they are not on the Nurse Prescribers' List). Any additional pain relief that they might provide can be at the cost of *increased side-effects caused by the opioid component* (constipation, in particular).

> When prescribing aspirin or paracetamol it is important to make sure that the patient is not already taking an aspirin- or a paracetamol-containing preparation (possibly bought over-the-counter).

Aspirin

Aspirin is indicated for mild to moderate pain including headache, transient musculoskeletal pain, and dysmenorrhoea; it has anti-inflammatory properties that may be useful, and is an antipyretic. The main side-effect is gastric irritation; rarely, gastric bleeding can be a serious complication. Aspirin increases bleeding time and must **not** be prescribed as an analgesic to patients receiving anticoagulants such as warfarin. Aspirin is also associated with bronchospasm and allergic reactions, particularly in patients with asthma. It should **not** be prescribed for patients with a history of hypersensitivity to aspirin or any other non-steroidal anti-inflammatory drug (NSAID)—which includes those in whom asthma, angioedema, urticaria or rhinitis have been precipitated by aspirin or another NSAID. Aspirin should **not** be prescribed for children and adolescents **under the age of 16 years** owing to its association with Reye's syndrome.

> **Other uses**
> Since aspirin decreases platelet aggregation, it is prescribed in low doses (e.g. 75–150 mg daily) to prevent cerebrovascular or cardiovascular disease. Aspirin is also *occasionally* prescribed for rheumatic conditions. Community Practitioner nurse prescribers should **not** prescribe aspirin for these conditions.

█ ASPIRIN

Indications   mild to moderate pain, pyrexia

Cautions   asthma, allergic disease, impaired hepatic or renal function (avoid if severe; see BNF appendixes 2 and 3), dehydration; preferably avoid during fever or viral infection in adolescents (risk of Reye's syndrome, see below); pregnancy (see BNF Appendix 4); elderly;

G6PD-deficiency (acceptable in a dose of up to 1 g daily in most G6PD-deficient individuals); concomitant use of drugs that increase risk of bleeding; **interactions**: see BNF Appendix 1 (aspirin)

Contra-indications   children under 16 years and in breast-feeding (Reye's syndrome—see below and BNF Appendix 5); previous or active peptic ulceration, haemophilia; not for treatment of gout

Hypersensitivity. Aspirin and other NSAIDs are **contra-indicated** in patients with a history of hypersensitivity to aspirin or any other NSAID—*which includes those* in whom attacks of *asthma, angioedema, urticaria or rhinitis* have been precipitated by aspirin or any other NSAID

Reye's Syndrome. Owing to an association with Reye's syndrome, the CSM has advised that aspirin-containing preparations should not be given to children under 16 years, unless specifically indicated, e.g. for Kawasaki syndrome.

Side-effects   generally mild and infrequent but high incidence of gastro-intestinal irritation with slight asymptomatic blood loss, increased bleeding time, bronchospasm and skin reactions in hypersensitive patients

Dose

- Usual, 300–600 mg every 4–6 hours when necessary, not more than 2.4 g daily without doctor's advice; CHILD under 16 years not recommended (see Reye's syndrome above)

◢*Prescribe as:*

¹**Dispersible Aspirin Tablets 300 mg** [PoM]
    Dispersible tablets, aspirin 300 mg. Net price 20 = £1.14
    Cautionary label added by pharmacist: dissolve or mix with water before taking and take with or after food

1. Nurse prescribers should prescribe packs containing no more than **32 tablets**, a max. of **3** packs of 32 tablets may be prescribed on each occasion: [PoM] but may be sold to the public under certain circumstances—for details see *Medicines, Ethics and Practice*, No. 33, London, Pharmaceutical Press, 2009 (and subsequent editions as available)

Ibuprofen

In single doses **ibuprofen** has analgesic activity comparable to that of paracetamol, but paracetamol is preferred for the management of pain, particularly in the elderly. Ibuprofen also has antipyretic properties. In regular dosage ibuprofen has a lasting analgesic and anti-inflammatory effect which makes it particularly useful for the treatment of pain associated with inflammation.

Like aspirin, ibuprofen has been associated with bronchospasm and allergic disorders; it is contra-indicated in patients with a history of hypersensitivity to aspirin or any other NSAID—which includes those in whom attacks of asthma, angioedema, urticaria or rhinitis have been precipitated by aspirin or any other NSAID.

The side-effects of ibuprofen include gastro-intestinal discomfort, nausea, diarrhoea, and occasionally bleeding and ulceration occur.

> **Other uses**
> Ibuprofen is prescribed for chronic inflammatory diseases. However, Community Practitioner nurse prescribers should not prescribe ibuprofen for indications or at doses other than those listed below.

◢ IBUPROFEN

Indications rheumatic and muscular pain, headache, dental pain, feverishness, symptoms of colds and influenza; in adults also backache, neuralgia, migraine, dysmenorrhoea

Cautions pregnancy and breast-feeding (see BNF Appendixes 4 and 5); allergic disorders (see Hypersensitivity below); coagulation defects; renal, cardiac or hepatic impairment (risk of deterioration of renal function—see also BNF Appendixes 2 and 3), elderly (risk of serious side-effects); **interactions**: see BNF Appendix 1 (NSAIDs)

Contra-indications previous or active peptic ulceration, severe heart failure

Hypersensitivity Contra-indicated in patients with a history of hypersensitivity to aspirin or any other NSAID—*which includes those* in whom attacks of *asthma, angioedema, urticaria, or rhinitis* have been precipitated by aspirin or any other NSAID

Side-effects gastro-intestinal discomfort including pain, indigestion and nausea; gastro-intestinal bleeding, bruising, bronchospasm, rashes, oedema, raised blood pressure, renal impairment; blood disorders reported; see BNF section 10.1.1 for other side-effects

Dose

- Initially 400 mg, then 200–400 mg every 4 hours, max. 1.2 g daily; if symptoms persist for more than 3 days refer to doctor
- Fever and pain in children, CHILD over 3 months and over 5 kg body-weight, 20–30 mg/kg daily in divided doses *or* 3–6 months 50 mg 3 times daily for max. 24 hours; 6–12 months 50 mg 3–4 times daily; 1–3 years 100 mg 3 times daily; 4–6 years 150 mg 3 times daily; 7–9 years 200 mg 3 times daily; 10–12 years 300 mg 3 times daily; refer to doctor if symptoms persist for more than 24 hours in child under 6 months or more than 3 days in child over 6 months
- Post-immunisation pyrexia, CHILD over 3 months 50 mg followed if necessary by second dose of 50 mg after 6 hours; if pyrexia persists refer to doctor

◢ *Prescribe as:*

¹Ibuprofen [PoM]

Tablets, coated, ibuprofen 200 mg, net price 16 = 32p

Oral suspension, ibuprofen 100 mg/5 mL, net price 100 mL = £1.47

Note Sugar-free versions are available and can be ordered by specifying 'sugar-free' on the prescription

Cautionary label added by pharmacist: take with or after food

1. May be sold to the public under certain circumstances—for details see *Medicines, Ethics and Practice*, No. 33, London, Pharmaceutical Press, 2009 (and subsequent editions as available)
Community Practitioner nurse prescribers should not prescribe outside the indications and doses above, other indications and doses are [PoM]

◢ PARACETAMOL

Indications mild to moderate pain, pyrexia

Cautions hepatic or renal impairment (see BNF Appendixes 2 and 3), alcohol dependence; **interactions**: see BNF Appendix 1 (paracetamol)

Side-effects side-effects rare, but rashes and blood disorders (including thrombocytopenia, leucopenia, neutropenia) reported; **important**: liver damage (and less frequently renal damage) following **overdosage**, immediate transfer to hospital essential

Dose

- 0.5–1 g every 4–6 hours; max. 4 g daily; CHILD 3 months–1 year 60–120 mg; 1–5 years 120–250 mg; 6–12 years 250–500 mg; these doses may be repeated every 4–6 hours when necessary; max. 4 doses in 24 hours
- Post-immunisation pyrexia, CHILD 2–3 months, 60 mg followed, if necessary, by second dose after 6 hours; if pyrexia persists refer to doctor

◢ *Prescribe as:*

¹Paracetamol Tablets 500 mg [PoM]

Tablets, paracetamol 500 mg, net price 16 = 17p, 32 = £1.18

Cautionary label added by pharmacist: Do not take more than 2 tablets at any one time. Do not take more than 8 in 24 hours. Do not take with any other paracetamol products

1. Nurse prescribers should prescribe packs containing no more than **32 tablets**, a max. of **3** packs of 32 tablets may be prescribed on each occasion: [PoM] but may be sold to the public under certain circumstances—for details see *Medicines, Ethics and Practice*, No. 33, London, Pharmaceutical Press, 2009 (and subsequent editions as available)

¹Soluble Paracetamol Tablets 500 mg [PoM]

Soluble tablets (Dispersible tablets), paracetamol 500 mg, net price 20 = £1.65

Cautionary label added by pharmacist: Do not take more than 2 tablets at any one time, do not take more than 8 in 24 hours, dissolve in water. Do not take with any other paracetamol products

1. Nurse prescribers should prescribe packs containing no more than **32 tablets**, a max. of **3** packs of 32 tablets may be prescribed on each occasion: [PoM] but may be sold to the public under certain circumstances—for details see *Medicines, Ethics and Practice*, No. 33, London, Pharmaceutical Press, 2009 (and subsequent editions as available)

Soluble Paracetamol Tablets 120 mg

Tablets (= Paediatric dispersible tablets), paracetamol 120 mg, net price 16-tab pack = 89p

Cautionary label added by pharmacist: Dissolve or mix with water before taking. Do not take with any other paracetamol products

---

Paracetamol

Paracetamol is similar in efficacy to aspirin, but has no demonstrable anti-inflammatory activity. It is less irritant to the stomach and for that reason paracetamol is now generally preferred to aspirin, particularly in the elderly. It must be remembered, however, that overdosage with paracetamol (alone or as an ingredient of a combination product) is particularly dangerous.

Paracetamol Oral Suspension 120 mg/5 mL

Oral suspension (= Paediatric mixture), paracetamol 120 mg/5 mL, net price 100 mL = 42p

Note Sugar-free version can be ordered by specifying 'sugar-free' on the prescription

Cautionary label added by pharmacist: Do not take with any other paracetamol products. If a 60-mg dose is required the pharmacist will supply an oral syringe and advise on how to give a 2.5-mL dose

Paracetamol Oral Suspension 250 mg/5 mL
   Oral suspension, (= Mixture) paracetamol 250 mg/
   5 mL, net price 100 mL = 66p
   Note Sugar-free version can be ordered by specifying 'sugar-free'
   on the prescription
   Cautionary label added by pharmacist: Do not take with any other
   paracetamol products.

Local anaesthetics

Corresponds to BNF section 15.2.

Lidocaine

Lidocaine (lignocaine) is effectively absorbed from mucous membranes and is a useful surface anaesthetic in concentrations of up to 10%. Except for surface anaesthesia, solutions should not usually exceed 1% in strength.

▌ LIDOCAINE HYDROCHLORIDE
   (Lignocaine Hydrochloride)

Indications surface anaesthesia (**important**: consult with doctor), see notes above

Cautions absorbed through mucosa therefore special care if history of epilepsy, cardiac disease, respiratory disease, hepatic or renal impairment, myasthenia gravis, or acute porphyria (BNF section 9.8.2) and in pregnancy; do **not** use in mouth (risk of choking); also **special care** in infants or young children

Side-effects include confusion, convulsions, respiratory depression, and cardiac depressant effects; allergic reactions (rarely anaphylaxis)

Administration see under preparations

◢Prescribe as:
Lidocaine Ointment
   Ointment, lidocaine hydrochloride 5% in a water-miscible basis. Net price 15 g = 88p.
   Administration sore nipples from breast-feeding, apply using
   gauze and wash off immediately before feed

Lidocaine and Chlorhexidine Gel
   Gel in disposable syringe, lidocaine hydrochloride 2%, chlorhexidine gluconate solution 0.25%, in a sterile lubricant basis in disposable syringe. Net price 6-mL syringe = £1.41, 11-mL syringe = £1.58. *Proprietary product: Instillagel* (6 mL, 11 mL)
   Administration into urethra, 6–11 mL

Prevention of neural tube defects

Corresponds to BNF section 9.1.2.

Prevention of neural tube defects

Folic acid supplements taken before and during pregnancy can reduce the occurrence of neural tube defects. The risk of a neural tube defect occurring in a child should be assessed and folic acid given as follows:

Women at a low risk of conceiving a child with a neural tube defect should be advised to take folic acid as a medicinal or food supplement at a dose of 400 micrograms daily before conception and until week 12 of pregnancy. Women who have not been taking folic acid and who suspect they are pregnant should start at once and continue until week 12 of pregnancy.

Couples are at a high risk of conceiving a child with a neural tube defect if either partner has a neural tube defect (or either partner has a family history of neural tube defects), if they have had a previous pregnancy affected by a neural tube defect, or if the woman has coeliac disease (or other malabsorption state), diabetes mellitus, sickle-cell anaemia, or is taking antiepileptic medicines (see also BNF section 4.8.1).

Women in the high-risk group who wish to become pregnant (or who are at risk of becoming pregnant) should be referred to a doctor because a higher dose of folic acid is appropriate.

 FOLIC ACID

Indications prevention of neural tube defects, see notes above

Dose

• See notes above

◢*Prescribe as:*

¹**Folic Acid Tablets, 400 micrograms**
Tablets, folic acid 400 micrograms, net price 90-tab pack = £2.32. *Proprietary product: Preconceive and possibly others*

1. Can be sold to the public provided daily doses do not exceed 500 micrograms

¹**Folic Acid Oral Solution 400 micrograms/5 mL**
Oral solution, folic acid 400 micrograms/5 mL, net price 150 mL = £1.40. *Proprietary product: Folicare*

1. Can be sold to the public provided daily doses do not exceed 500 micrograms

Nicotine replacement therapy

Corresponds to BNF section 4.10

Smoking cessation interventions are a cost-effective way of reducing ill health and prolonging life. Smokers should be advised to stop and offered help if interested in doing so, with follow-up where appropriate.

Where possible, smokers should have access to a smoking cessation clinic for behavioural support **Nicotine replacement therapy** is an effective aid to smoking cessation for those smoking more than 10 cigarettes a day. The form of nicotine replacement therapy chosen should take into account individual preference and tolerance of side-effects. Smokers who are pregnant or breast-feeding should discuss the use of nicotine replacement therapy with a healthcare professional trained in smoking cessation; nicotine replacement therapy should be used only if other measures have failed.

Cigarette smoking should stop completely before starting nicotine replacement therapy. If complete smoking cessation is not possible some nicotine preparations are licensed for use as part of a programme to reduce smoking before stopping completely; the smoking cessation regimen can be followed during a quit attempt.

Nicotine replacement therapy should be prescribed for short durations at a time and the prescriptions repeated only if the smoker demonstrates a continuing attempt to stop smoking (see also NICE guidance, BNF section 4.10).

Cross-references to the BNF are provided but nurse prescribers may only prescribe those items that are listed on the Nurse Prescribers' List.

■ **NICOTINE**

Indications adjunct to smoking cessation

Cautions severe or unstable cardiovascular disease (including hospitalisation for severe arrhythmias, recent myocardial infarction, or recent cerebrovascular accident)—initiate under medical supervision; uncontrolled hyperthyroidism; diabetes mellitus (monitor blood-glucose concentration closely when initiating treatment); phaeochromocytoma; *oral preparations*, oesophagitis, gastritis, peptic ulcers; *patches*, skin disorders (patches should not be placed on broken skin); hepatic impairment (see BNF Appendix 2); renal impairment (see BNF Appendix 3); pregnancy (see BNF Appendix 4); breast-feeding (see BNF Appendix 5)
Note Most warnings under Cautions also apply to continuation of cigarette smoking

Side-effects gastro-intestinal disturbances (including nausea, vomiting, dyspepsia); headache, dizziness; influenza-like symptoms; dry mouth; rash; *less frequently* palpitation; *rarely* atrial fibrillation; *with nasal spray*, sneezing, epistaxis, watering eyes, ear sensations; *with lozenges*, thirst, paraesthesia of mouth, taste disturbances; *with patches*, skin reactions (discontinue if severe)—vasculitis also reported, blood pressure changes; *with patches or lozenges*, sleep disturbances, nightmares, chest pain; *with gum or lozenges*, mouth ulceration, increased salivation; *with gum, lozenge,* *sublingual tablets*, or *inhalation cartridges*, hiccups, throat irritation

Dose

- See under preparations, below

◢***Prescribe as:***

¹**Nicotine Inhalation Cartridge for Oromucosal Use**

Cartridge (for oromucosal use), nicotine 10 mg, net price 6-cartridge (starter) pack = £4.46, 42-cartridge (refill) pack = £14.02. *Proprietary products: Nicorette Inhalator*

Administration Smoking cessation, ADULT and CHILD over 12 years, inhale when urge to smoke occurs; initially use 6–12 cartridges daily for up to 8 weeks, then reduce number of cartridges used by half over next 2 weeks and then stop altogether after further 2 weeks; review treatment if abstinence not achieved in 3 months

Smoking reduction, ADULT and CHILD over 12 years, inhale when urge to smoke occurs between smoking episodes; reduce smoking within 6 weeks and attempt smoking cessation within 6 months; review treatment if abstinence not achieved within 9 months

Note Children under 18 years should consult a healthcare professional before starting a smoking-reduction regimen

1. For use with an inhalation mouthpiece; starter pack contains 6 cartridges with inhalator device and holder, refill pack contains 42 cartridges with inhalator device

Nicotine Lozenge

Lozenge, sugar-free, nicotine (as bitartrate) 1 mg, net price pack of 12 = £1.71, pack of 36 = £4.27, pack of 96 = £9.12; 2 mg, pack of 12 = £1.99, pack of 36 = £4.95, pack of 96 = £10.60 (*proprietary product: Nicotinell Mint Lozenge*) or nicotine (as resinate complex) 1.5mg, net price pack of 12 = £1.68, pack of 36 = £4.18, pack of 96 = £8.94 (*proprietary product: Nicopass Lozenge*) or nicotine (as polacrilex) 2 mg, net price pack of 36 = £5.12, pack of 72 = £9.97, 4 mg pack of 36 = £5.12, pack of 72 = £9.97 (*proprietary product: NiQuitin Lozenge*)

Excipients include aspartame (BNF section 9.4.1)

Dose Smoking cessation, initially suck 1 lozenge every 1–2 hours, when urge to smoke occurs; max. 30 mg daily for lozenges of 1 mg, 1.5 mg, 2 mg, or 60 mg daily for lozenges of 4 mg; withdraw gradually after 3 months; max. period of treatment should not usually exceed 6 months (may vary between brands, see BNF); CHILD 12–18 years, withdraw gradually and review treatment if abstinence not achieved within 3 months

Smoking reduction (*NiQuitin* lozenges), suck 1 lozenge when urge to smoke occurs between smoking episodes (max. 15 lozenges daily); reduce smoking within 6 weeks and attempt cessation within 6 months; review treatment if abstinence not achieved within 9 months

Temporary abstinence (*NiQuitin* lozenges), suck 1 lozenge every 1–2 hours when urge to smoke occurs between smoking episodes (max. 15 lozenges daily); review treatment if unable to undertake permanent quit attempt within 6 months

Note Children under 18 years should consult a healthcare professional before starting smoking-reduction regimen. *Nicotinell* or *Nicopass* lozenges should not be given to children under 18 years without doctor's advice. *Nicopass* lozenges should not be given to patients heavily dependent on nicotine

Nicotine Sublingual Tablets

Sublingual tablet, nicotine (as a cyclodextrin complex) 2 mg, net price starter pack of 2 × 15-tablet discs with dispenser = £4.46, refill pack of 7 × 15-tablet discs = £12.04. *Proprietary product: Nicorette Microtab*

Dose Smoking cessation, individuals smoking 20 cigarettes or fewer daily, sublingually, 2 mg each hour; for patients who fail to stop smoking or have significant withdrawal symptoms, consider increasing to 4 mg each hour

Individuals smoking more than 20 cigarettes daily, sublingually, 4 mg each hour

Max. 80 mg daily; treatment should be continued for at least 3 months followed by a gradual reduction in dosage; review treatment if abstinence not achieved within 9 months, CHILD 12–18 years, treatment continued for up to 8 weeks followed by gradual reduction over 4 weeks; review treatment if abstinence not achieved within 3 months

Nicotine Medicated Chewing Gum

Chewing gum, sugar-free, nicotine 2 mg, net price pack of 12 = £1.71, pack of 15 = £1.71, pack of 24 = £2.85, pack of 30 = £3.25, pack of 96 = £8.26, pack of 105 = £8.89; 4 mg, net price pack of 12 = £1.70, pack of 15 = £2.11, pack of 24 = £2.85, pack of 30 = £3.99, pack of 96 = £8.55, pack of 105 = £10.83, pack of 204 = £14.23. *Proprietary products: Nicorette Gum, Nicotinell Gum, NiQuitin Gum*

Note Available in various flavours

Dose Smoking cessation, individuals smoking 20 cigarettes or fewer daily, initially one 2-mg piece chewed slowly (chew gum until taste becomes strong, then rest gum between cheek and gum, when taste fades start chewing again) for approx. 30 minutes, when urge to smoke occurs; individuals smoking more than 20 cigarettes daily or needing more than 15 pieces of 2-mg gum daily may need 4-mg strength; max. 15 pieces of 4-mg strength daily; withdraw gradually after 3 months; max. period of treatment should not exceed 6 months (may vary between brands, see BNF) CHILD 12–18 years, withdraw gradually and review treatment if abstinence not achieved within 3 months

Smoking reduction (*Nicorette* and *NiQuitin* gums), chew one piece when urge to smoke occurs between smoking episodes; reduce smoking within 6 weeks and attempt smoking cessation within 6 months; review treatment if abstinence not achieved within 9 months

Temporary abstinence (*NiQuitin* gum), chew 1 piece when urge to smoke occurs between smoking episodes (max. 15 pieces daily); review treatment if unable to undertake permanent quit attempt within 6 months

Note Children under 18 years should consult a healthcare professional before starting a smoking-reduction regimen

Nicotine Nasal Spray

Nasal spray, nicotine 500 micrograms/metered spray, net price 200-spray unit = £13.30. *Proprietary product: Nicorette Nasal Spray*

Administration Smoking cessation, ADULT and CHILD over 12 years, apply 1 spray into each nostril as required to max. twice an hour for 16 hours daily (max. 64 sprays daily) for 8 weeks, then reduce gradually over next 4 weeks (reduce by half at end of first 2 weeks, stop altogether after further 2 weeks); review treatment if abstinence not achieved within 3 months

¹**Nicotine Transdermal Patches**

Patches, self-adhesive, releasing in each 16 hours, nicotine approx. 5 mg, 10 mg, or 15 mg (*proprietary product: Boots NicAssist Patch, Nicorette Patch*) or releasing in each 24 hours nicotine approx. 7 mg, 14 mg, or 21 mg (*proprietary products: Nicopatch, Nicotinell TTS, NiQuitin*)

Note For pack sizes and prices, see individual products in BNF section 4.10

Administration see individual products in BNF section 4.10

1. Prescriber should specify the brand to be dispensed

Drugs for the mouth

Corresponds to BNF sections 12.3.2, 12.3.1, 12.3.4 and 12.3.5

Candida albicans may cause thrush and other forms of stomatitis which sometimes follow the use of broad-spectrum antibacterials or cytotoxics; withdrawal of the causative drug may lead to rapid resolution; alternatively antifungal treatment may be required. Infants may develop thrush which responds to use of an antifungal mouth preparation.

Patients with denture stomatitis may also respond to the use of an antifungal mouth preparation. They should be instructed to cleanse their dentures thoroughly to prevent reinfection; ideally they should leave their dentures out as often as possible during the treatment period. Proper dental appraisal may be necessary.

> Patients with an unexplained mouth ulcer of more than 3 weeks' duration require urgent referral to exclude oral cancer.

Oral antifungal drugs

Miconazole and **nystatin** are suitable for the treatment of oral thrush.

■ MICONAZOLE

Indications prevention and treatment of oral fungal infections

Cautions pregnancy (see BNF Appendix 4) and breast-feeding; avoid in acute porphyria (BNF section 9.8.2); **interactions**: see BNF Appendix 1 (antifungals, imidazole); oral gel may be absorbed enough for interactions to occur after application to the oral mucosa

Contra-indications hepatic impairment; impaired swallowing reflex in infants; first 6 months of life of an infant born preterm

Side-effects nausea, vomiting; rash; *very rarely* diarrhoea (usually on long-term treatment), hepatitis, toxic epidermal necrolysis, and Stevens-Johnson syndrome

Dose
• See under preparation

▲*Prescribe as:*
¹**Miconazole Oromucosal Gel** ⃞PoM⃞
   Oral gel, sugar-free, orange-flavoured, miconazole 24 mg/mL (20 mg/g). Net price 15-g tube = £2.84, 80-g tube = £4.47. *Proprietary product: Daktarin Oral Gel*
   Dose place 5–10 mL in the mouth after food 4 times daily; retain near oral lesions before swallowing; CHILD 4 months–2 years 2.5 mL twice daily, smeared around the mouth; 2–6 years 5 mL twice daily, retained near lesions before swallowing; over 6 years 5 mL 4 times daily, retained near lesions before swallowing; treatment continued for 48 hours after lesions have healed
   Localised lesions, smear small amount of gel on affected area with clean finger 4 times daily for 5–7 days (dentures should be removed at night and brushed with gel); treatment continued for 48 hours after lesions have healed (prescribe 15-g tube)
   Note Not licensed for use in children under 4 months of age or during first 6 months of life of an infant born preterm
   1. 15-g tube can be sold to public

■ NYSTATIN

Indications oral and perioral fungal infections

Side-effects oral irritation and sensitisation, nausea reported; see also BNF section 5.2

Dose
• See under preparation, below

▲*Prescribe as:*
Nystatin Oral Suspension ⃞PoM⃞
   Oral suspension, nystatin 100 000 units/mL. Net price 30 mL (with pipette) = £1.91. *Proprietary product: Nystan Oral Suspension*
   Dose ADULT and CHILD over 1 month, place 1 mL in the mouth after food and retain near the lesions 4 times daily, usually for 7 days (continued for 48 hours after lesions have resolved); NEONATE [unlicensed], place 1 mL in the mouth 4 times daily after feeds, usually for 7 days (continued for 48 hours after lesions have healed)
   Note Not licensed for treating candidiasis in NEONATE under 1 month but the Department of Health has advised that a Community Practitioner Nurse Prescriber may prescribe nystatin oral suspension for a NEONATE, at the dose stated above, provided that there is a clear diagnosis of oral thrush. The nurse prescriber must only prescribe within their own competence and must accept clinical and medicolegal responsibility for prescribing
   Only medical practitioners should prescribe for immunosuppressed patients

Thymol

Mouthwashes have a mechanical cleansing action. **Mouthwash solution-tablets** may contain thymol as well as an antimicrobial; they are used to remove unpleasant tastes.

■ THYMOL

Indications oral hygiene, see notes above

Dose
• See under preparation, below

▲*Prescribe as:*
Mouthwash Solution-tablets
   Tablets, may contain antimicrobial, colouring, and flavouring agents in a suitable soluble effervescent basis to make a mouthwash. Net price, 100 = £15.02
   Dose Dissolve 1 tablet in a glass of warm water and rinse
   Note Mouthwash Solution-tablets may contain ingredients such as thymol

Drugs for oral ulceration and inflammation

Choline salicylate dental gel has some analgesic action and may provide relief for recurrent mouth ulcers, but excessive application or confinement under a denture irritates the mucosa and can itself cause ulceration. Choline salicylate dental gel should no longer be used for teething or in children under 16 years, because of the theoretical risk of Reye's syndrome.

> Patients with an unexplained mouth ulcer of more than 3 weeks' duration require urgent referral to exclude oral cancer.

◼ SALICYLATES

Indications mild oral and perioral lesions

Cautions not to be applied to dentures—leave at least 30 minutes before re-insertion of dentures; frequent application, especially in children, may give rise to salicylate poisoning

Contra-indications children under 16 years
Reye's syndrome The CHM has advised (April 2009) that topical oral pain relief products containing salicylate salts should not be used in children under 16 years, as a cautionary measure due to the theoretical risk of Reye's syndrome

Dose
- ADULT and CHILD over 16 years, apply ½-inch of gel with gentle massage not more often than every 3 hours

◢ *Prescribe as:*
Choline Salicylate Dental Gel
  Oral gel, choline salicylate 8.7% in a flavoured gel basis, net price 15 g = £1.89. *Proprietary product: Bonjela* (sugar-free)

Treatment of dry mouth

Dry mouth may be relieved in many patients by simple measures such as frequent sips of cool drinks or sucking pieces of ice or sugar-free fruit pastilles. Sugar-free chewing gum stimulates salivation in patients with residual salivary function.

Saliva stimulating tablets may be prescribed for dry mouth in patients with salivary gland impairment (and patent salivary ducts).

◢ *Prescribe as:*
Saliva Stimulating Tablets
  Tablets, sugar-free, citric acid, malic acid and other ingredients in a sorbitol base, net price 100-tab pack = £4.86. *Proprietary product: SST tablets*
  Dose symptomatic treatment of dry mouth in patients with impaired salivary gland function and patent salivary ducts, allow 1 tablet to dissolve slowly in the mouth when required

Removal of earwax

Corresponds to BNF section 12.1.3

Wax is a normal bodily secretion which provides a protective film on the meatal skin and need only be removed if it causes deafness or interferes with a proper view of the ear drum. Ear irrigation is generally best avoided in young children and in patients with a history of recurring otitis externa, a history of ear drum perforation, or previous ear surgery. A person who has hearing only in one ear should not have that ear irrigated because even a very slight risk of damage is unacceptable in this situation.

Wax may be removed by irrigation with water (warmed to body temperature). If necessary, wax can be softened with simple remedies such as **olive oil** ear drops or **almond oil** ear drops. **Sodium bicarbonate** ear drops are also effective but may cause dryness of the ear canal. If the wax is hard and impacted, the drops may be used twice daily for a few days before irrigation; otherwise the wax may be softened on the day of irrigation. The patient should lie with the affected ear uppermost for 5 to 10 minutes after a generous amount of the softening remedy has been introduced into the ear.

> Cross references to the BNF are provided but nurse prescribers may only prescribe those items that are listed on the Nurse Prescribers' List.

◢ *Prescribe as:*
Almond Oil Ear Drops
  Ear drops, almond oil in a suitable container
  Administration allow to warm to room temperature and use as indicated above
  Note Do not heat

Olive Oil Ear Drops
  Ear drops, olive oil in a suitable container
  Administration allow to warm to room temperature and use as indicated above
  Note Do not heat

Sodium Bicarbonate Ear Drops
  Ear drops, sodium bicarbonate 5%. Net price 10 mL = £1.25
  Administration allow to warm to room temperature and use as indicated above

Drugs for threadworms

Corresponds to BNF section 5.5.1.

Anthelmintics are effective for threadworm infections (enterobiasis) but their use needs to be combined with hygiene measures to break the cycle of auto-infection. Threadworms are highly infectious therefore all members of the family need to be treated at the same time.

Adult threadworms do not live for longer than 6 weeks; eggs need to be swallowed and subjected to the action of digestive juices for the development of the worms. Direct multiplication of worms does not take place in the large bowel. Adult females lay eggs on the perianal skin, which causes pruritus. Scratching the area leads to eggs being transmitted on fingers to the mouth, often via food eaten with unwashed hands. It is therefore important to advise patients to wash their hands and scrub their nails before each meal and after each visit to the toilet. A bath taken immediately after rising will remove eggs laid during the night. Advice for patients is included in the packaging of most preparations, but it is useful to reinforce this advice verbally.

> Mebendazole and piperazine are also prescribed for other infections (e.g. roundworms). Community Practitioner nurse prescribers should, however, prescribe them for threadworm infection **only.**

Mebendazole

Mebendazole is the drug of choice for patients over 2 years of age with threadworms. It is given as a single dose but as reinfection is very common, a second dose may be given after 2 weeks.

▊ MEBENDAZOLE

Indications   threadworm infection; other infections, on doctor's prescription only

Cautions   pregnancy (toxicity found in *rats*), see package insert information below; breast-feeding (see BNF Appendix 5); **interactions**: BNF Appendix 1 (mebendazole)

Side-effects   *very rarely* abdominal pain, diarrhoea, convulsions (in infants) and rash (including Stevens-Johnson syndrome and toxic epidermal necrolysis)

Dose

● Threadworms, ADULT and CHILD over 2 years, 100 mg as a single dose; if reinfection occurs second dose may be needed after 2 weeks; CHILD under 2 years not recommended

◢*Prescribe as:*

¹Mebendazole Tablets 100 mg [PoM]

Tablets, chewable, mebendazole 100 mg. Net price 6-tab pack = £1.36.

Note The package insert includes the information that the tablets are not suitable for women known to be pregnant or for children under 2 years

1. Packs containing no more than 800 mg and labelled to show a max. single dose of 100 mg are on sale to the public for the treatment of threadworm infection in adults and children over 2 years

¹Mebendazole Oral Suspension 100 mg/5 mL [PoM]

Oral Suspension, mebendazole 100 mg/5 mL. Net price 30 mL = £1.59. *Proprietary product:* Vermox

Note The package insert includes the information that the suspension is not suitable for women known to be pregnant or for children under 2 years

1. Packs containing no more than 800 mg and labelled to show a max. single dose of 100 mg are on sale to the public for the treatment of threadworm infection in adults and children over 2 years

Piperazine

Piperazine is available in combination with sennosides; 2 doses are given for threadworm infection with an interval of 2 weeks between them.

▊ PIPERAZINE

Indications   threadworm infection; other infections, on doctor's prescription only

Cautions   renal impairment (avoid if severe—see BNF Appendix 3), liver impairment (BNF Appendix 2); epilepsy, pregnancy (see below for warnings in packs and BNF Appendix 4); breast-feeding (BNF Appendix 5)

Side-effects   nausea, vomiting, colic, diarrhoea; allergic reactions including urticaria, bronchospasm, and rare reports of arthralgia, fever, Stevens-Johnson syndrome and angioedema; rarely dizziness, muscular incoordination ('worm wobble'); drowsiness, nystagmus, vertigo, blurred vision, confusion and clonic contractions in patients with neurological or renal abnormalities

Dose

● Threadworms, see under preparation, below

◢*Prescribe as:*

For cautions, contra-indications, and side-effects of Senna, see p. 8

Piperazine and Senna Powder

Oral powder, piperazine phosphate 4 g, total sennosides (calculated as sennoside B) 15.3 mg/sachet. Net price 2-dose sachet pack = £1.73. *Proprietary product:* Pripsen

Dose   stirred into a small glass of milk or water and drunk immediately, ADULT and CHILD over 6 years, content of 1 sachet as a single dose (bedtime in adults or morning in children), repeated after 14 days; CHILD 3 months–1 year, 1 level 2.5-mL spoonful in the morning, repeated after 14 days; CHILD 1–6 years, 1 level 5-mL spoonful in the morning, repeated after 14 days

Cautionary label added by pharmacist: dissolve or mix with water before taking

Note For children under 10 years, only one dual-dose treatment should be given in any 28-day period without medical advice.

Packs on sale to the public carry a warning to avoid in epilepsy, in liver or kidney disease, and to seek medical advice in pregnancy

Drugs for scabies and head lice

Corresponds to BNF section 13.10.4

Scabies

Permethrin is used for the treatment of *scabies* (*Sarcoptes scabiei*); **malathion** can be used if permethrin is not appropriate.

The following should be noted:

- *alcoholic lotions* are not recommended (owing to irritation of excoriated skin and genitalia);
- it is not necessary to apply preparations *after a hot bath* (a hot bath may even increase absorption into the blood, removing the drug from its site of action on the skin).

All members of the affected household should be treated simultaneously. Treatment should be applied to the whole body including the scalp, neck, face, and ears. Particular attention should be paid to the webs of the fingers and toes, and lotion brushed under the ends of the nails. It is now recommended that malathion and permethrin should be applied twice, one week apart. Patients with hyperkeratotic (crusted or 'Norwegian') scabies may require 2 or 3 applications of acaricide on consecutive days to ensure that enough penetrates the skin crusts to kill all the mites.

It is important to warn users to reapply treatment to the hands if they are washed.

The itch of scabies persists for some weeks after the infestation has been eliminated and antipruritic treatment may be required. Application of **crotamiton** can be used to control itching after treatment with more effective acaricides, but caution is necessary if the skin is excoriated.

> Cross references to the BNF are provided but nurse prescribers may only prescribe those items that are listed on the Nurse Prescribers' List.

Head lice

Malathion, and the **pyrethroid**, phenothrin, can be used against head lice (*Pediculus humanus capitis*) but lice in some districts have developed resistance, resistance to two or more parasiticidal preparations has also been reported. Careful application of **dimeticone**, which acts on the surface of head lice, is also effective.

Head lice infestation (pediculosis) should be treated with lotion or liquid preparations. Shampoos are diluted too much in use to be effective. Aqueous formulations are preferred in severe eczema, and for patients with asthma, and small children, to avoid alcoholic fumes. A contact time of 12 hours or overnight treatment is recommended for lotions and liquids. A 2-hour treatment is not sufficient to kill eggs.

In general, a course of treatment for head lice should be 2 applications of product 7 days apart to prevent lice emerging from any eggs that survive the first application.

The policy of rotating insecticides on a district-wide basis is now considered outmoded. To overcome the development of resistance, a mosaic strategy is required whereby, if a course of treatment fails to cure, a different insecticide is used for the next course. If a course of treatment with phenothrin fails, then a non-pyrethroid parasiticidal product should be used for the next course.

Wet combing methods Head lice may be mechanically removed by combing wet hair meticulously with a plastic detection comb (probably for at least 30 minutes each time) over the whole scalp at 4-day intervals for a minimum of 2 weeks; hair conditioner can be used to facilitate the process. Several products are available and some are prescribable on the NHS, including *Bug Buster kit, Full Marks Solution, Lyclear Spray Away, Nitcomb-M2, Nitcomb-S1, Nitlotion, Nitty Gritty NitFree* (consult Drug Tariff—see Appliances and Reagents (p. 4) for links to online Drug Tariffs).

> Not all preparations included here are licensed for *crab lice* therefore advice on crab lice has not been included

> Individuals can rarely react to certain ingredients in preparations applied to the skin. Special care is required when prescribing skin and scalp products for these individuals—see BNF section 13.1.3. Excipients associated with sensitisation are shown under individual product entries

Dimeticone

Dimeticone coats head lice and interferes with water balance in lice by preventing the excretion of water; it is less active against eggs and treatment should be repeated after 7 days.

◢ DIMETICONE

Indications head lice
Cautions avoid contact with eyes; children under 6 months, medical supervision required
Side-effects skin irritation
Administration rub into dry hair and scalp, allow to dry naturally, shampoo after minimum 8 hours (or overnight); repeat application after 7 days

◢Prescribe as:
Dimeticone Lotion 4%
Lotion, dimeticone 4%, net price 50 mL = £2.98, 120-mL spray pack = £7.13, 150 mL = £6.83. *Proprietary product: Hedrin*
Note Patients should be told to keep hair away from fire and flames during treatment

Malathion

Malathion is recommended for *scabies* and *head lice* (for details see notes above).

The risk of systemic effects associated with 1–2 applications of malathion is considered to be very low; however applications of lotions repeated at intervals of less than 1 week *or* application for more than 3 consecutive weeks should be **avoided** since the likelihood of eradication of lice is not increased.

◢ MALATHION

Indications scabies, head lice

Cautions avoid contact with eyes; do not use on broken or secondarily infected skin; do not use more than once a week for 3 consecutive weeks; use in children under 6 months on doctor's advice only

Side-effects skin irritation and hypersensitivity reactions; chemical burns also reported

Administration head lice, rub into dry hair and scalp, allow to dry naturally, remove by washing 12 hours later (see also notes above); repeat application after 7 days

Scabies, apply over whole body, wash off after 24 hours; if hands are washed with soap within 24 hours, they should be retreated; see also notes above; repeat application after 7 days

Note For scabies, manufacturer recommends application to the body but not necessarily to the head and neck. However, application should be extended to the scalp, neck, face, and ears.

◢*Prescribe as:*

Malathion Aqueous Lotion 0.5%

Aqueous lotion, malathion 0.5% in an aqueous basis. *Proprietary products: Derbac-M Liquid* (net price 50 mL = £2.27, 200 mL = £5.70), *Quellada M* (50 mL = £1.85, 200 mL = £4.62)

Excipients include cetostearyl alcohol, fragrance, hydroxybenzoates (parabens)

Permethrin

Permethrin is effective for *scabies* (for details see notes above). Permethrin is active against *head lice* but the formulation and licensed methods of application of the current products make them unsuitable for the treatment of head lice.

◢ PERMETHRIN

Indications scabies

Cautions avoid contact with eyes; do not use on broken or secondarily infected skin; use for scabies in children under 2 years on doctor's advice only

Side-effects pruritus, erythema, and stinging; rarely rashes and oedema

Administration scabies, apply over whole body and wash off after 8–12 hours; CHILD (see also Cautions above) apply over whole body including face, neck, scalp, and ears; cream should be reapplied to hands if they are washed with soap and water within 8 hours of application (see notes above); repeat application after 7 days

Note Manufacturer recommends application to the body but to exclude the head and neck. However, application should be extended to the scalp, neck, face, and ears.

Larger patients may require up to two 30-g packs for adequate treatment

◢*Prescribe as:*

Permethrin Cream 5%

Cream, permethrin 5%. Net price 30 g = £5.71. *Proprietary product: Lyclear Dermal Cream*

Excipients may include butylated hydroxytoluene, wool fat derivative

Phenothrin

Phenothrin is recommended for *head lice* (for details see notes above).

◢ PHENOTHRIN

Indications head lice

Cautions avoid contact with eyes; do not use on broken or secondarily infected skin; do not use more than once a week for 3 weeks at a time; use for children under 6 months on doctor's advice only

Side-effects skin irritation

Administration head lice, apply to dry hair, allow to dry naturally; shampoo after 12 hours or next day, comb hair while still wet; repeat application after 7 days

◢*Prescribe as:*

Phenothrin Aqueous Lotion

Liquid, phenothrin 0.5% in an aqueous basis. Net price 200 mL = £6.27. *Proprietary product: Full Marks Liquid*

Excipients include cetostearyl alcohol, fragrance, hydroxybenzoates (parabens)

Skin preparations

Emollients

Corresponds to BNF section 13.2.1 and 13.2.1.1.

Emollients soothe, smooth and hydrate the skin and are indicated for all dry or scaling disorders. Their effects are short-lived and they should be applied frequently even after improvement occurs. They are useful in dry and eczematous disorders, and to a lesser extent in psoriasis. Light emollients such as **aqueous cream** are suitable for many patients with dry skin but a wide range of more greasy preparations including **white soft paraffin**, **emulsifying ointment**, and **liquid and white soft paraffin ointment** are available; the severity of the condition, patient preference and site of application will often guide the choice of emollient; emollients should be applied in the direction of hair growth. Ointments may exacerbate acne and folliculitis. Some ingredients may occasionally cause sensitisation (BNF section 13.1.3) and this should be suspected if an eczematous reaction occurs.

> **Fire hazard with paraffin-based emollients**
> Emulsifying ointment *or* 50% Liquid Paraffin and 50% White Soft Paraffin Ointment in contact with dressings and clothing is easily ignited by a naked flame. The risk will be greater when these preparations are applied to large areas of the body, and clothing or dressings become soaked with the ointment. Patients should be told to keep away from fire or flames, and not to smoke when using these preparations. The risk of fire should be considered when using large quantities of any paraffin-based emollient.

Preparations such as **aqueous cream** and **emulsifying ointment** can be used as soap substitutes for hand washing and in the bath; the preparation is rubbed on the skin before rinsing off completely. The addition of a bath oil may also be helpful; several proprietary emollient bath additives are available (see below).

Arachis oil (peanut oil) is occasionally used for cleansing in dry skin conditions.

> Individuals can rarely react to certain ingredients in preparations applied to the skin. Special care is required when prescribing skin and scalp products for these individuals—see BNF section 13.1.3. Excipients associated with sensitisation are shown under individual product entries

EMOLLIENTS

◢*Prescribe as:*

Aqueous Cream
 Cream, emulsifying ointment 30%, [1]phenoxyethanol 1%, in freshly boiled and cooled purified water. Net price 100 g = 70p, 500 g = £1.70
 Excipients include cetostearyl alcohol

1. The BP permits use of alternative antimicrobials provided their identity and concentration are stated on the label

Emulsifying Ointment
 Ointment, emulsifying wax 30%, white soft paraffin 50%, liquid paraffin 20%. Net price 500 g = £2.15
 Excipients include cetostearyl alcohol

Hydrous Ointment
 (Also known as Oily Cream)
 Ointment, dried magnesium sulphate 0.5%, phenoxyethanol 1%, wool alcohols ointment 50% in freshly boiled and cooled purified water. Net price 500 g = £2.18

Liquid and White Soft Paraffin Ointment
 Ointment, liquid paraffin 50%, white soft paraffin 50%. Net price 500 g = £3.94

Paraffin, White Soft
 White petroleum jelly. Net price 100 g = 46p

Paraffin, Yellow Soft
 Yellow petroleum jelly. Net price 100 g = 38p

◢**Proprietary emollients,** *prescribe as:*
Cetraben® Emollient Cream (Genus)
 Cream, white soft paraffin 13.2%, light liquid paraffin 10.5%. Net price 50-g pump pack = £1.17, 150-g pump pack = £2.88, 500-g pump pack = £5.39, 1.05-kg pump pack = £11.11
 Excipients include cetostearyl alcohol, hydroxybenzoates (parabens)
 For inflamed, damaged, dry or chapped skin including eczema

Dermamist® (Alliance)
 Spray application, white soft paraffin 10% in a basis containing liquid paraffin, fractionated coconut oil. Net price 250-mL pressurised aerosol unit = £6.45
 For dry skin conditions including eczema, ichthyosis, pruritus of the elderly
 Cautions flammable

Diprobase® Cream (Schering-Plough)
 Cream, cetomacrogol 2.25%, cetostearyl alcohol 7.2%, liquid paraffin 6%, white soft paraffin 15%, water-miscible basis. Net price 50 g = £1.30; 500-g pump pack = £6.58
 Excipients include cetostearyl alcohol, chlorocresol
 For dry skin conditions

Diprobase® Ointment (Schering-Plough)
 Ointment, liquid paraffin 5%, white soft paraffin 95%, basis. Net price 50 g = £1.30
 For dry skin conditions

Doublebase® (Dermal)
 Gel, isopropyl myristate 15%, liquid paraffin 15%, net price 100 g = £2.69; 500 g = £5.92
 For dry, chapped or itchy skin conditions

E45® Cream (Crookes)
 Cream, light liquid paraffin 12.6%, white soft paraffin 14.5%, hypoallergenic anhydrous wool fat (hypoallergenic lanolin) 1% in self-emulsifying monostearin. Net price 50 g = £1.40, 125 g = £2.25, 350 g = £4.46, 500-g pump pack = £5.39
 Excipients include cetyl alcohol, hydroxybenzoates (parabens)
 For dry skin conditions

Emollin® (C D Medical)
 Spray, liquid paraffin 50%, white soft paraffin 50% in aerosol basis, net price 150 mL = £3.74, 240 mL = £5.98
 For dry skin conditions

Epaderm® (Mölnlycke)
Ointment, emulsifying wax 30%, yellow soft paraffin 30%, liquid paraffin 40%, net price 125 g = £3.62, 500 g = £6.14, 1 kg = £11.44
Excipients include cetostearyl alcohol
For use as an emollient or soap substitute

Hydromol® Cream (Alliance)
Cream, sodium pidolate 2.5%, liquid paraffin 13.8%, net price 50 g = £2.04, 100 g = £3.80, 500 g = £11.09
Excipients include cetyl alcohol, hydroxybenzoates (parabens)
For dry skin conditions

Hydromol® Ointment (Ferndale)
Ointment, yellow soft paraffin 30%, emulsifying wax 30%, liquid paraffin 40%, net price 125 g = £2.79, 500 g = £4.74
Excipients include cetostearyl alcohol
For use as an emollient bath additive, or soap substitute

Linola® Gamma Cream (Linderma)
Cream, evening primrose oil 20%, net price 50 g = £2.83, 250 g = £8.20
Excipients include beeswax, hydroxybenzoates (parabens), propylene glycol
Cautions epilepsy (but hazard unlikely with topical preparations)
For dry skin conditions

Lipobase® (Astellas)
Cream, fatty cream basis. Net price 50 g = £2.08
Excipients include cetostearyl alcohol, hydroxybenzoates (parabens)
For dry skin conditions

Neutrogena® Norwegian Formula Dermatological Cream (J&J)
Cream, glycerol 40% in an emollient basis. Net price 100 g = £3.77
Excipients include cetostearyl alcohol, hydroxybenzoates (parabens)
For dry skin conditions

Oilatum® Cream (Stiefel)
Cream, light liquid paraffin 6%, white soft paraffin 15%. Net price 40 g = £1.30, 150 g = £2.46, 500-mL pump pack = £4.99, 1.05-litre pump pack = £9.98
Excipients include benzyl alcohol, cetostearyl alcohol
For dry skin conditions

Oilatum® Junior Cream (Stiefel)
Cream, light liquid paraffin 6%, white soft paraffin 15%, net price 150 g = £3.38, 350 mL = £4.65, 500 mL = £4.99, 1.05-litre pump pack = £9.98
Excipients include benzyl alcohol, cetostearyl alcohol
For dry skin conditions

QV® Cream (Crawford)
Cream, glycerol 10%, light liquid paraffin 10%, white soft paraffin 5%, net price 100 g = £1.95, 500 g = £5.60
Excipients include cetostearyl alcohol, hydroxybenzoates (parabens)
For dry skin conditions including eczema, psoriasis, ichthyosis, pruritus

QV® Lotion (Crawford)
Lotion, white soft paraffin 5%, net price 250 mL = £3.00
Excipients include cetostearyl alcohol, hydroxybenzoates (parabens)
For dry skin conditions including eczema, psoriasis, ichthyosis, pruritus

QV® Wash (Crawford)
Wash, glycerol 10%, net price 200 mL = £2.50
Excipients include hydroxybenzoates (parabens)
For dry skin conditions including eczema, psoriasis, ichthyosis, and pruritus, use as soap substitute

Ultrabase® (Valeant)
Cream, water-miscible, containing liquid paraffin and white soft paraffin. Net price 50 g = 89p; 500-g pump pack = £6.44
Excipients include fragrance, hydroxybenzoates (parabens), disodium edetate, stearyl alcohol
For dry skin conditions

Unguentum M® (Almirall)
Cream, saturated neutral oil, liquid paraffin, white soft paraffin. Net price 50 g = £1.41, 100 g = £2.78, 200-mL pump pack = £5.50, 500 g = £8.48
Excipients include cetostearyl alcohol, polysorbate 40, propylene glycol, sorbic acid
For dry skin conditions and nappy rash

Zerobase® Cream (Zeroderma)
Cream, liquid paraffin 11%, net price 500-g pump pack = £5.99
Excipients include cetostearyl alcohol, chlorocresol
For dry skin conditions

◢ Proprietary emollient bath additives, *prescribe as:*

¹**Balneum®** (Almirall)
Bath oil, soya oil 84.75%. Net price 200 mL = £2.48, 500 mL = £5.38, 1 litre = £10.39
Excipients include butylated hydroxytoluene, propylene glycol, fragrance
For dry skin conditions including those associated with dermatitis and eczema; add 20–60 mL/bath (INFANT 5–15 mL); do not use undiluted

1. Some pack sizes may not be prescribed on the NHS and are not listed here

Cetraben® Emollient Bath Additive (Genus)
Emollient bath additive, light liquid paraffin 82.8%, net price 500 mL = £5.25
For dry skin conditions, including eczema, add 1–2 capfuls/bath (CHILD 0.5–1 capful) or apply to wet skin and rinse

Dermalo® (Dermal)
Bath emollient, acetylated wool alcohols 5%, liquid paraffin 65%. Net price 500 mL = £3.50
For dermatitis, dry skin conditions including ichthyosis and pruritus of the elderly; add 15–20 mL/bath (INFANT and CHILD 5–10 mL) or apply to wet skin and rinse

Diprobath® (Schering-Plough)
Bath additive, isopropyl myristate 39%, light liquid paraffin 46%. Net price 500 mL = £6.84
For dry skin conditions including dermatitis and eczema; add 25–50 mL/bath (INFANT 10 mL); do not use undiluted

Doublebase® Emollient Bath Additive (Dermal)
Emollient bath additive, liquid paraffin 65%, net price 500 mL = £5.54
Excipients include cetostearyl alcohol
For dry skin conditions including dermatitis, ichthyosis, and pruritus of the elderly; add 15–20 mL/bath, (INFANT and CHILD 5–10 mL)

Doublebase® Emollient Shower Gel (Dermal)
Emollient Shower Gel, isopropyl myristate 15%, liquid paraffin 15%. Net price 200 g = £5.29
For dry, chapped or itchy skin conditions

Doublebase® Emollient Wash Gel (Dermal)
Emollient Wash Gel, isopropyl myristate 15%, liquid paraffin 15%. Net price 200-g pump pack = £5.29
For dry, chapped, or itchy skin conditions

Hydromol® Bath and Shower Emollient (Alliance)

Bath and Shower Emollient, isopropyl myristate 13%, light liquid paraffin 37.8%. Net price 350 mL = £3.61, 500 mL = £4.11, 1 litre = £8.19

For dry skin conditions including eczema, ichthyosis and pruritus of the elderly; add 1–3 capfuls/bath (INFANT 0.5–2 capfuls) or apply to wet skin and rinse

Imuderm® Bath Oil (Goldshield)

Bath oil, almond oil 30%, light liquid paraffin 69.6%, net price 250 mL = £3.75

Excipients include butylated hydroxyanisole

For dry skin conditions including dermatitis, eczema, pruritus of the elderly and ichthyosis, add 15–30 mL/bath (INFANT and CHILD 7.5–15 mL) or rub into dry skin until absorbed

Oilatum® Emollient (Stiefel)

Bath additive (emulsion), acetylated wool alcohols 5%, liquid paraffin 63.4%. Net price 250 mL = £2.75; 500 mL = £4.57

Excipients include isopropyl palmitate, fragrance

For dry skin conditions including dermatitis, pruritus of the elderly and ichthyosis; add 1–3 capfuls/bath (INFANT 0.5–2 capfuls) or apply to wet skin and rinse

Oilatum® Junior Emollient Bath Additive (Stiefel)

Bath additive, light liquid paraffin 63.4%, net price 150 mL = £2.82, 250 mL = £3.25, 300 mL = £5.10, 500 mL = £5.75

Excipients include wool fat, isopropyl palmitate

For dry skin conditions including dermatitis, pruritus of the elderly and ichthyosis; add 1–3 capfuls/bath (INFANT 0.5–2 capfuls) or apply to wet skin and rinse

Oilatum® Gel (Stiefel)

Shower emollient (gel), light liquid paraffin 70%. Net price 150 g = £5.15

Excipients include fragrance

For dry skin conditions including dermatitis

QV® Bath Oil (Crawford)

Bath oil, light liquid paraffin 85.09%, net price 200 mL = £2.20, 500 mL = £4.50

Excipients include hydroxybenzoates (parabens)

For dry skin conditions including eczema, ichthyosis, and pruritus of the elderly, add 10 mL/bath (CHILD 7 mL, INFANT 4 mL) or apply to wet skin and rinse

---

Barrier preparations

Corresponds to BNF section 13.2.2.

Barrier preparations often contain water-repellent substances such as **dimeticone** (dimethicone) or other silicones. They are used on the skin around stomas, bedsores, and pressure areas in the elderly where the skin is intact. Where the skin has broken down, barrier preparations have a limited role in protecting adjacent skin. They are no substitute for adequate nursing care and it is doubtful if they are any more effective than the traditional compound **zinc ointments**. A spray preparation, **zinc oxide and dimeticone spray**, is also available.

Nappy rash Barrier creams and ointments are used for protection against nappy rash which is usually a local dermatitis. The first line of treatment is to ensure that nappies are changed frequently and that tightly fitting water-proof pants are avoided. The rash may clear when left exposed to the air, and a barrier preparation may be helpful. If the rash is associated with a fungal infection, an antifungal cream such as clotrimazole cream is useful.

▌ DIMETICONE (SILICONE)

Dimeticone barrier creams containing at least 10%

◀*Prescribe as:*

Dimeticone Cream (*Conotrane*)

Cream, benzalkonium chloride 0.1%, dimeticone '350' 22%. Net price 100 g = 88p; 500 g = £3.51.

Excipients include cetostearyl alcohol, fragrance

For nappy and urinary rash and pressure sores

Dimeticone Cream (*Siopel*)

Barrier cream, dimeticone '1000' 10%, cetrimide 0.3%, arachis (peanut) oil. Net price 50 g = £2.15.

Excipients include butylated hydroxytoluene, cetostearyl alcohol, hydroxybenzoates (parabens)

For protection against water-soluble irritants

Dimeticone Cream (*Vasogen*)

Barrier cream, dimeticone 20%, calamine 1.5%, zinc oxide 7.5%. Net price 50 g = 80p; 100 g = £1.36.

Excipients include hydroxybenzoates (parabens), wool fat

For nappy rash, pressure sores, ileostomy and colostomy care

▌ TITANIUM or ZINC

◀*Prescribe as:*

Titanium Ointment

Ointment, titanium dioxide 20%, titanium peroxide 5%, titanium salicylate 3% in a basis containing dimeticone, light liquid paraffin, white soft paraffin, and benzoin tincture. Net price 30 g = £2.01. *Proprietary product: Metanium Ointment*

For nappy rash

Zinc Cream

Cream, zinc oxide 32%, arachis (peanut) oil 32%, calcium hydroxide 0.045%, oleic acid 0.5%, wool fat 8%, in freshly boiled and cooled purified water, net price 50 g = 50p.

For nappy and urinary rash and eczematous conditions

Zinc Ointment

Ointment, zinc oxide 15%, in Simple Ointment BP 1988 (which contains wool fat 5%, hard paraffin 5%, cetostearyl alcohol 5%, white soft paraffin 85%), net price 25 g = 22p.

For nappy and urinary rash and eczematous conditions

Zinc and Castor Oil Ointment

Ointment, zinc oxide 7.5%, castor oil 50%, arachis (peanut) oil 30.5%, white beeswax 10%, cetostearyl alcohol 2%. Net price 100 g = 70p.

For nappy and urinary rash

Zinc Oxide and Dimeticone Spray

Spray application, dimeticone 1.04%, zinc oxide 12.5%, in a basis containing wool alcohols, cetostearyl alcohol, white soft paraffin, liquid paraffin, dextran, propellants. Net price 115-g pressurised aerosol unit = £3.54. *Proprietary product: Sprilon*

Excipients include cetostearyl alcohol, hydroxybenzoates (parabens), wool fat

For urinary rash, pressure sores, leg ulcers, moist eczema, fissures, fistulae and ileostomy care

Cautions flammable

Pruritus

Corresponds to BNF section 13.3.

Pruritus may be caused by systemic disease (such as drug hypersensitivity, obstructive jaundice, endocrine disease, and certain malignant diseases), skin disease (e.g. psoriasis, eczema, urticaria, and scabies), or as a side-effect of opioid analgesics. Where possible the underlying causes should be treated. An **emollient** may be of value where the pruritus is associated with dry skin (which is common in otherwise healthy elderly people).

Preparations containing **crotamiton** are sometimes used in pruritus but are of uncertain value. Crotamiton can be used to control itching after treatment with a parasiticidal preparation for scabies (see p. 19).

Preparations containing calamine are often ineffective and therefore these preparations are no longer included in the NPF.

◼ CROTAMITON

Indications pruritus (including pruritus after scabies); see notes above

Cautions avoid use near eyes and broken skin; use on doctor's advice for children under 3 years

Contra-indications acute exudative dermatoses

Administration pruritus, apply 2–3 times daily; CHILD below 3 years, apply once daily

◢*Prescribe as:*
Crotamiton Cream 10%
Cream, crotamiton 10%. Net price 30 g = £2.27; 100 g = £3.95
Excipients include beeswax, fragrance, hydroxybenzoates (parabens), stearyl alcohol

Crotamiton Lotion 10%
Lotion, crotamiton 10%. Net price 100 mL = £2.99
Excipients include cetyl alcohol, fragrance, propylene glycol, sorbic acid, stearyl alcohol

Fungal infections

Corresponds to BNF section 13.10.2.

Fungal skin infections can be prevented by keeping the susceptible area as clean and dry as possible. Localised fungal infections such as ringworm infection and candidal skin infection can be treated with **clotrimazole cream**, **econazole cream** or **miconazole cream**.

To prevent relapse, local antifungal treatment should be continued for 1–2 weeks after the disappearance of all signs of infection. Systemic antifungal therapy is necessary for nail or scalp infection or if the skin infection is widespread, disseminated, or intractable.

◼ CLOTRIMAZOLE

Indications fungal skin infections

Cautions avoid contact with eyes and mucous membranes

Side-effects occasional skin irritation or hypersensitivity reactions including mild burning sensation, erythema, and itching (discontinue if severe)

Administration apply 2–3 times daily

◢*Prescribe as:*
Clotrimazole Cream 1%
Cream, clotrimazole 1%. Net price 20 g = £1.84
Excipients are not shown because preparation available from several sources; for sensitised individuals, check that product dispensed is free from any sensitising ingredient

◼ ECONAZOLE NITRATE

Indications see under Clotrimazole
Cautions see under Clotrimazole
Side-effects see under Clotrimazole
Administration apply twice daily

◢*Prescribe as:*
Econazole Cream 1%
Cream, econazole nitrate 1%. *Proprietary products: Ecostatin® Cream* (net price 15 g = £1.49, 30 g = £2.75), *Pevaryl® Cream* (net price 30 g = £2.65)
Excipients include butylated hydroxyanisole, fragrance

◼ MICONAZOLE NITRATE

Indications see under Clotrimazole
Cautions see under Clotrimazole
Side-effects see under Clotrimazole
Administration apply twice daily continuing for 10 days after lesions have healed

◢*Prescribe as:*
Miconazole Cream 2%
Cream, miconazole nitrate 2%. Net price 20 g = £2.05, 45 g = £1.97
Excipients are not shown because preparation available from several sources; for sensitised individuals, check that product dispensed is free from any sensitising ingredient

Boils

Boils are generally treated with a systemic antibacterial, but **magnesium sulphate paste** can be used as an adjunct when dressing the boil or carbuncle.

◼ MAGNESIUM SULPHATE

Indications paste used as an adjunct in the management of boils

Administration apply under dressing

◢*Prescribe as:*
Magnesium Sulphate Paste
Paste, dried magnesium sulphate 45 g, glycerol 55 g, phenol 500 mg. Net price 25 g = 70p, 50 g = 81p
Note Stir before use

Disinfection and cleansing

Corresponds to BNF section 13.11.

Physiological saline

Sterile **sodium chloride solution** 0.9% is suitable for general cleansing of skin and wounds but tap water is often appropriate.

■ SODIUM CHLORIDE

Indications skin cleansing

◢*Prescribe as:*

Sterile Sodium Chloride Solution 0.9%

Sterile solution, sodium chloride 0.9%. To be used undiluted for topical irrigation of wounds.

Aerosol can: 100-mL can = £1.94 (*proprietary product: Stericlens*); 200-mL can = £2.65 (*proprietary product: Nine Lives*); 240-mL can = £2.95 (*proprietary products: Stericlens, Irriclens*)

Bellows Pack: 120-mL = £1.53 (*proprietary product: Flowfusor*)

Bottle: 30 × 45-mL = £13.20, 30 × 100-mL = £19.50 (*proprietary product: MiniVersol*); 500 mL = 70p, 1 litre = 80p (*proprietary products include: Versol*)

Sachets and pods: 25 × 20-mL unit = £5.50 (*proprietary products include: Irripod, Steripod*); 25 × 25-mL sachet = £6.10 (*proprietary product: Normasol*); 10 × 100-mL sachet = £7.41 (*proprietary product: Normasol*); other sizes also prescribable if available

Chlorhexidine

Chlorhexidine gluconate aqueous and alcoholic solutions are useful where skin disinfection is required.

■ CHLORHEXIDINE

Indications skin disinfection

Cautions avoid contact with eyes, brain, meninges and middle ear; not for use in body cavities; alcoholic solutions not suitable before diathermy

Side-effects occasional sensitivity

◢*Prescribe as:*

Chlorhexidine Gluconate Alcoholic Solution

Solution, chlorhexidine gluconate solution 2.5% (≡chlorhexidine gluconate 0.5%), in an alcoholic solution, net price 600 mL (clear) = £2.06; 600 mL (pink) = £2.06, 200-mL spray = £1.77, 500-mL spray = £3.01; 600 mL (blue) = £2.25. *Proprietary products: Hydrex Solution, Hydrex Spray*

Note Flammable

Chlorhexidine Gluconate Alcoholic Solution

Cutaneous solution, sterile, chlorhexidine gluconate 2% in isopropyl alcohol 70%, net price (single applicator) 0.67 mL = 30p, 1.5 mL = 55p, 3 mL = 85p, 10.5 mL = £2.92, 26 mL = £6.50. *Proprietary product: ChloraPrep*

For skin disinfection before invasive procedures; CHILD under 2 months, not recommended

Note Flammable

Chlorhexidine Gluconate Aqueous Solution

Solution, (sterile), pink, chlorhexidine gluconate 0.05%, net price 25 × 25-mL sachet = £5.40; 10 × 100-mL sachet = £6.67. *Proprietary product: Unisept*

Povidone–iodine

Povidone–iodine aqueous solution 10% is useful where skin disinfection is required.

■ POVIDONE–IODINE

Indications skin disinfection

Cautions pregnancy (BNF Appendix 4), breast-feeding (BNF Appendix 5), broken skin (see below), renal impairment (avoid regular application to inflamed or broken skin or mucosa)

Large open wounds The application of povidone–iodine to large wounds or severe burns may produce systemic adverse effects such as metabolic acidosis, hypernatraemia and impairment of renal function

Contra-indications preterm neonate gestational age under 32 weeks; avoid regular use in patients with thyroid disorders or those receiving lithium therapy

Side-effects rarely sensitivity; may interfere with thyroid function tests

◢*Prescribe as:*

Povidone–Iodine Solution 10%

Solution, povidone–iodine 10% in aqueous solution. Net price 500 mL = £2.50. *Proprietary product: Videne Antiseptic Solution.*

Administration apply undiluted in pre-operative skin disinfection and general antisepsis; NEONATE not recommended for regular use (and contra-indicated if body-weight below 1.5 kg)

Note. Not for body cavity irrigation

Wound management products and elasticated garments

See BNF Appendix 8

Wound management products and elasticated garments described as ⟨NHS⟩ in the BNF are not in the Drug Tariff or on the Nurse Prescribers' List.

Medicated bandages and stocking

Corresponds to BNF Appendix 8.

Zinc Paste Bandage has been used with compression bandaging for the treatment of venous leg ulcers. However, paste bandages are associated with hypersensitivity reactions and should be used with caution.

Zinc paste bandages are also used with **coal tar** or **ichthammol** in chronic lichenified skin conditions such as chronic eczema (ichthammol often being preferred since its action is considered to be milder). They are also used with **calamine** in milder eczematous skin conditions.

 ZINC OXIDE

Indications see notes above
Administration see notes above and under preparations below

◢*Prescribe as:*
Zinc Paste Bandage, BP 1993
Cotton fabric, plain weave, impregnated with suitable paste containing zinc oxide; requires additional bandaging. Net price 6 m × 7.5 cm = £3.23. *Proprietary product: Viscopaste PB7* (10%), *excipients: include* cetostearyl alcohol, hydroxybenzoates

Zinc Paste and Calamine Bandage
(Drug Tariff specification 5).
Cotton fabric, plain weave, impregnated with suitable paste containing calamine and zinc oxide; requires additional bandaging. Net price 6 m × 7.5 cm = £3.33. *Proprietary product: Calaband*

Zinc Paste and Ichthammol Bandage, BP 1993
Cotton fabric, plain weave, impregnated with suitable paste containing zinc oxide and ichthammol; requires additional bandaging. Net price 6 m × 7.5 cm = £3.31. *Proprietary product: Ichthopaste* (6/2%), *excipients: include* cetostearyl alcohol
Uses see BNF section 13.5

Zinc Oxide Impregnated Medicated Bandage
Cotton fabric, selvedge weave, impregnated with paste containing zinc oxide 15%. Net price 6 m × 7.5 cm = £3.24. *Proprietary product: Steripaste*
Excipients include polysorbate 80

Zinc Oxide Impregnated Medicated Stocking
Stocking, sterile rayon, impregnated with ointment containing zinc oxide 20%. Net price 4-pouch carton = £12.52; 10-pouch carton = £31.30. *Proprietary product: Zipzoc*
Administration chronic leg ulcers; can be used under appropriate compression bandages or hosiery in chronic venous insufficiency

Peak flow meters

Corresponds to BNF section 3.1.5

Measurement of peak flow is particularly helpful for patients who are 'poor perceivers' and hence slow to detect deterioration in their asthma, and for those with moderate or severe asthma.

Standard-range peak flow meters are suitable for both adults and children; low-range peak flow meters are appropriate for severely restricted airflow in adults and children. Patients must be given clear guidance on the action they should take if the peak flow falls below a specified level.

◢*Prescribe as:*
Standard-range peak flow meter
   Conforms to standard EN 13826
   Peak flow meter, range 60–800 litres/minute (*Proprietary products include: MicroPeak,* net price = £6.50; *Mini-Wright,* £6.86; *Personal Best,* £6.48; *Pocketpeak,* £6.53); range 50–800 litres/minute (*Proprietary product: Vitalograph,* £4.50, children's coloured version also available); range 15–999 litres/minute (*Proprietary product: Piko-1,* £9.50); also replacement mouthpieces available (not interchangeable between brands)
   Note Readings from new peak flow meters are often lower than those obtained from old Wright-scale peak flow meters and the correct chart should be used

Low-range peak flow meter
   Conforms to standard EN 13826 except for scale range
   Peak flow meter, range 30–400 litres/minute, net price = £6.90 (*proprietary product: Mini-Wright*), 50–400 litres/minute = £6.53 (*proprietary product: Pocketpeak*); also replacement mouthpieces available (not interchangeable between brands)
   Note Readings from new peak flow meters are often lower than those obtained from old Wright-scale peak flow meters and the correct chart should be used

Urinary catheters and appliances

Urinary appliances

These are listed in Part IXB of the Drug Tariff (Part 5 of the Scottish Drug Tariff, Part III of the Northern Ireland Drug Tariff).

> For links to the online Drug Tariffs, see Appliances and Reagents p. 4

Urethral catheters

These are listed in Part IXA of the Drug Tariff (Part 3 of the Scottish Drug Tariff, Part III of the Northern Ireland Drug Tariff).

Maintenance of indwelling urinary catheters

Corresponds to BNF section 7.4.4.

The deposition which occurs on urinary catheters is usually chiefly composed of phosphate and to minimise this, the catheter (if latex) should be changed at least as often as every 6 weeks. If the catheter is to be left for longer periods a silicone catheter should be used together with the appropriate use of catheter maintenance solutions. Repeated blockage usually indicates that the catheter needs to be changed.

▉ CATHETER PATENCY SOLUTIONS

Indications   catheter care; see also under preparations, below

Administration   to be warmed to body temperature and instilled as required, see also under preparations, below

◀*Prescribe as:*
Chlorhexidine 0.02% Catheter Maintenance Solution

Sterile solution, chlorhexidine 0.02%. *Proprietary product: Uro-Tainer Chlorhexidine* (net price 100-mL sachet = £2.60)

For mechanical cleansing; discontinue if burning or haematuria occur

Sodium Chloride 0.9% Catheter Maintenance Solution

Sterile solution, sodium chloride 0.9%. *Proprietary products: OptiFlo S* (Net price 50- and 100-mL sachets = £3.20), *Uriflex S* (100-mL sachet = £2.40) *Uro-Tainer Sodium Chloride* (50- and 100-mL sachets = £3.23)

For removal of clots and other debris, to be instilled as required

'Solution G' Catheter Maintenance Solution

Sterile solution, citric acid 3.23%, magnesium oxide 0.38%, sodium bicarbonate 0.7%, disodium edetate 0.01%. *Proprietary products: OptiFlo G* (Net price 50- and 100-mL sachets = £3.40), *Uriflex G* (100-mL sachet = £2.40); *Uro-Tainer Twin Suby G* (2 × 30 mL = £4.42)

For prevention of catheter encrustation and crystallisation; in very severe cases use 'Solution R'

'Solution R' Catheter Maintenance Solution

Sterile solution, citric acid 6%, gluconolactone 0.6%, magnesium carbonate 2.8%, disodium edetate 0.01%. *Proprietary products: OptiFlo R* (Net price 50- and 100-mL sachets = £3.40), *Uriflex R* (100-mL sachet = £2.40), *Uro-Tainer Twin Solutio R* (2 × 30 mL = £4.42)

For prevention of catheter encrustation and dissolution of crystallisation if 'Solution G' unsuccessful

Water

Corresponds to BNF section 9.2.2.1

◀*Prescribe as:*
Water for Injections [PoM]

Net price 1-mL amp = 18p; 2-mL amp = 18p; 5-mL amp = 33p; 10-mL amp = 33p; 20-mL amp = 92p; 50-mL amp = £1.91; 100-mL vial = £2.07

Stoma care

Corresponds to BNF section 1.8—prescribing for patients with stoma

The 3 major types of abdominal stoma are:

- colostomy
- ileostomy
- urostomy

Each requires the collection of body waste into an artificial appliance (the 'bag') attached to the body. The bags and accessories are tailored for the different types of stoma.

Colostomy In a colostomy, a stoma is formed from a cut end of colon. The output depends on the position along the colon from which the stoma is created; the further down the colon's length from which the colostomy is formed, the greater the volume of fluid that can be reabsorbed. The discharge changes from a liquid or paste-like consistency to a nearly fully formed stool mass. The nature of the discharge determines whether the bag can be drainable or non-drainable.

A *permanent colostomy* is formed by surgical removal of the diseased part of the colon. A *temporary colostomy* may be created to allow a distal part of the colon to recover from trauma (e.g. a gunshot wound, stabbing, or road traffic accident). On healing, the colon is surgically rejoined to permit normal faecal output.

Ileostomy In an ileostomy, a piece of ileum is brought to the abdominal surface following removal of varying lengths of the colon:

- pan-procto colectomy—removal of all parts of the colon
- total colectomy—removal of all of the colon apart from the rectal stump. Later, it may be possible to create an artificial pouch in the abdominal cavity which rejoins the ileum to the rectal stump, permitting normal discharge of faeces.

Urostomy A urostomy (ileal conduit) is created by the diversion of the two ureters into a piece of colon or, more commonly, ileum. The piece of intestine is brought to the abdominal surface to form a stoma. Normal gastro-intestinal function is resumed after removal of the piece to form the stoma.

Stoma appliances

The only essential prerequisites for stoma management are the collection receptacle (the 'bag') and a means of attaching it to the abdominal wall. However, practical and successful management demands, and the *Drug Tariff* permits, the supply of a range of other components.

Stoma bags and flanges Modern stoma bags are oblong or tapered, rectangular, plastic receptacles. A circular opening is placed over the stoma. Around the opening is a flange that is used to attach the bag to the abdominal wall. A bag may be non-drainable, for use

with a descending colostomy with a solid and predictable action; or it may be drainable, having a wide-necked opening with a **bag closure**, for all other types of colostomy and for an ileostomy. A bag for a urostomy has a tap for regular drainage of urine.

A bag may be one- or two-piece, depending on whether the flange is integral with the bag, or separate.

The **flange** may be attached to the abdominal wall by double-sided adhesive rings, or by the separate use of plasters or other adhesives. Skin care is important in stoma management, and a varied range of karaya-based flanges is also available. Non-adhesive flanges are available for stomas that have a solid output only.

As a colostomy stoma is much larger than that formed from ileum, a range of flange sizes is available. However, most flanges have to be cut to size by the patient, for which measuring cards are commonly provided.

A **two-piece bag** is one in which the flange is separate from the bag, and from which the bag can be detached without removing the flange from the skin. The bag is clipped to the flange, and a waist belt can be clipped to the bag. The two-piece bag permits rapid changing should the bag develop a leak.

Accessories **Adhesive removers** are available to assist in cleaning the skin after the flange has been removed. Care must be taken to ensure that their use does not cause or aggravate skin soreness.

Bag covers of a wide range of designs and colours are available. They are particularly useful for bags that are made of transparent or semi-transparent material.

Belts are available for use with one- or two-piece bags. Their use may aid the confidence of wearers in the ability of the adhesive to keep the bag attached to the abdomen, and be necessary in wearers with irregularly shaped or distended abdomens.

Deodorants can be placed in the bag to minimise the odour from the discharge.

Filters are integral to many colostomy and ileostomy bags, and are useful for the removal of flatus from the bag. Replacement filters can be incorporated into some designs.

Irrigation/wash-out appliances are available for colostomy patients who evacuate the bowel once every 24 to 48 hours as an alternative to uncontrolled, irregular evacuation through the stoma. A cone-shaped irrigation system is inserted into the stoma, and the distal colon filled with 1–1.5 litres of warm water. Only replacement parts can be prescribed on the NHS; complete systems have to be supplied by a hospital.

Skin fillers and protectives comprise a range of aerosols, barrier creams, gels, lotions, pastes, and wipes. Fillers are used if the abdominal wall is distorted and needs levelling to allow successful attachment of the flange. Protectives are used in cases of skin soreness, but care must be taken to ensure that their use does not compromise the adhesiveness of the flange.

Stoma caps can be clipped to the flange of a two-piece bag for short periods (e.g. during swimming or sports). Their use is practicable only with colostomies that have regular faecal movements.

Tubing that may be prescribed consists of drainage tubing for urostomy bags, for use by immobile patients, or for overnight attachment to night drainage bags.

Prescribing medicines Prescribing for patients with stoma calls for special care. The following is a brief account of some of the main points to be borne in mind.

Enemas and washouts should **not** be prescribed for patients with an ileostomy as they may cause rapid and severe dehydration.

Colostomy patients may suffer from constipation and whenever possible should be treated by increasing fluid intake or dietary fibre. **Bulk-forming drugs** (see p. 6) should be tried. If they are insufficient, as small a dose as possible of senna (see Stimulant Laxatives, p. 7) should be used.

The doctor's advice should be obtained for other complications such as diarrhoea.

New patients are usually given advice about the use of *cleansing agents*, *protective creams*, *lotions*, *deodorants*, or *sealants* whilst in hospital, either by the surgeon or by stoma care nurses. Voluntary organisations offer help and support to patients with stoma.

Stoma appliances and associated products

These are listed in Part IXC of the Drug Tariff (Part 6 of the Scottish Drug Tariff, Part III of the Northern Ireland Drug Tariff).

Urostomy pouches

These are listed in Part IXC of the Drug Tariff (Part 6 of the Scottish Drug Tariff, Part III of the Northern Ireland Drug Tariff).

For links to online Drug Tariffs, see Appliances and Reagents p. 4

Appliances and reagents for diabetes

Hypodermic equipment

Corresponds to BNF section 6.1.1.3.

Patients should be advised on the safe disposal of lancets, single-use syringes, and needles. Suitable arrangements for the safe disposal of contaminated waste must be made before these products are prescribed for patients who are carriers of infectious diseases.

Lancets may be used on their own or in an automatic 'finger pricking' device such as *Autolet* or *Glucolet* . Various devices take different lancets; see BNF section 6.1.1.3 for further details.

■ HYPODERMIC EQUIPMENT

See BNF section 6.1.1.3

Hypodermic equipment described as NHS in the BNF are not in the Drug Tariff, or on the Nurse Prescribers' list.

Monitoring agents

Corresponds to BNF section 6.1.6.

Glucose (for glucose tolerance test) is **not** on the Nurse Prescribers' List.

■ URINALYSIS

Urine testing for glucose is useful in patients who find blood glucose monitoring difficult. Tests for glucose employ reagent strips specific to glucose; *Clinistix* is suitable for screening purposes only.

Reagents are also available to test for ketones and protein in urine but these are usually used in clinics; patients are rarely required to do these tests themselves unless they become unwell.

◢ Reagents

See BNF section 6.1.6

Reagents described as NHS in the BNF are not in the Drug Tariff, or on the Nurse Prescribers' List.

■ BLOOD GLUCOSE MONITORING

Blood glucose monitoring using a meter gives a direct measure of the glucose concentration at the time of the test and can detect hypoglycaemia as well as hyperglycaemia. Patients should be properly trained in the use of blood glucose monitoring systems and the appropriate action to take, based on the results obtained. Inadequate understanding of the normal fluctuations in blood glucose can lead to confusion and inappropriate action.

Note In the UK blood glucose concentration is expressed in mmol/litre and Diabetes UK advises that these units should be used for self-monitoring of blood glucose. In other European countries units of mg/100 mL (or mg/dL) are commonly used.

It is advisable to check that the meter is pre-set in the correct units.

◢ Reagents

See BNF section 6.1.6

Reagents described as NHS in the BNF are not in the Drug Tariff, or on the Nurse Prescribers' List.

Eye-drop dispensers

Eye-drop dispensers are available to aid the instillation of eye drops especially amongst the elderly, visually impaired, arthritic, or otherwise physically limited patients. Eye-drop dispensers are for use with plastic eye drop bottles, for repeat use by individual patients. Details of products available may be found in the Drug Tariff section IXA (Part 3 of the Scottish Drug Tariff, Part III of the Northern Ireland Drug Tariff).

For links to online Drug Tariffs, see Appliances and Reagents, p. 4

Fertility and gynaecological products

Polythene Ring Pessaries
Pessaries, 7.5 mm thick, 50–80 mm (rising in 3 mm), 80–100 mm (rising in 5 mm), and 110 mm. Net price 1 pessary = £1.90

Antiseptics phenols or cresols should be avoided because absorption may cause severe irritation; pessaries may be washed in soapy water or boiled

PVC Ring Pessaries
Pessaries, 1.25 cm thick, 50–80 mm (rising in 3 mm), 85–100 mm (rising in 5 mm), and 110 mm. Net price 1 pessary = £2.06

Antiseptics phenols or cresols should be avoided as these may be absorbed causing irritation in use

Contraceptive devices

Corresponds to BNF section 7.3.4

Intra-uterine devices

The intra-uterine device (IUD) is suitable for older parous women and as a second-line contraceptive in young nulliparous women who should be carefully screened because they have an increased background risk of pelvic inflammatory disease (see BNF section 7.3.4)

The healthcare professional inserting (or removing) the intra-uterine device should be fully trained in the technique and should provide full counselling backed by the patient information leaflet.

INTRA-UTERINE CONTRACEPTIVE DEVICES

Indications contraception, see BNF section 7.3.4

Cautions see BNF section 7.3.4; also anaemia, heavy menses (progestogen intra-uterine system might be preferable, BNF section 7.3.2.3), endometriosis, severe primary dysmenorrhoea, history of pelvic inflammatory disease, diabetes, fertility problems, nulliparity and young age, severely scarred uterus (including after endometrial resection) or severe cervical stenosis; valvular heart disease or history of endocarditis (see BNF section 5.1, Table 2); drug- or disease-induced immunosuppression (risk of infection—avoid if marked immunosuppression); epilepsy (risk of seizure at time of insertion); increased risk of expulsion if inserted before uterine involution; gynaecological examination before insertion, 6–8 weeks after, then annually but counsel women to see doctor promptly in case of significant symptoms, especially pain; anticoagulant therapy (avoid if possible); remove if pregnancy occurs; if pregnancy occurs, increased likelihood that it may be ectopic

Contra-indications pregnancy, severe anaemia, recent sexually transmitted infection (if not fully investigated and treated), unexplained uterine bleeding, distorted or small uterine cavity, genital malignancy, active trophoblastic disease (until return to normal of urine- and plasma-gonadotrophin concentration), pelvic inflammatory disease, established or marked immunosuppression; *copper devices:* copper allergy, Wilson's disease, medical diathermy

Side-effects uterine or cervical perforation, displacement, expulsion; pelvic infection may be exacerbated, menorrhagia, dysmenorrhoea, allergy; *on insertion*: pain (alleviated by NSAID such as oral ibuprofen, 30 minutes before insertion) and bleeding, occasionally epileptic seizure and vasovagal attack

◢*Prescribe as:*

Flexi-T® 300

Intra-uterine device, copper wire, surface area approx. 300 mm² wound on vertical stem of T-shaped plastic carrier, impregnated with barium sulphate for radio-opacity, monofilament thread attached to base of vertical stem; preloaded in inserter, net price = £9.47

For uterine length over 5 cm; replacement every 5 years (see also notes in BNF section 7.3.4)

Flexi-T® + 380

Intra-uterine device, copper wire, surface area approx. 380 mm² wound on vertical stem of T-shaped plastic carrier with copper sleeve on each arm, impregnated with barium sulphate for radio-opacity, monofilament thread attached to base of vertical stem; preloaded in inserter, net price = £10.06

For uterine length over 6 cm; replacement every 5 years (see also notes in BNF section 7.3.4)

GyneFix®

Intra-uterine device, 6 copper sleeves with surface area of 330 mm² on polypropylene thread, net price = £26.64

Suitable for all uterine sizes; replacement every 5 years; fitting technique requires additional training

Load® 375

Intra-uterine device, copper wire, surface area approx. 375 mm² wound on vertical stem of U-shaped plastic carrier, impregnated with barium sulphate for radio-opacity, monofilament thread attached to base of vertical stem; preloaded in inserter, net price = £8.00

For uterine length over 7 cm; replacement every 5 years (see also notes in BNF section 7.3.4)

Mini TT 380® Slimline

Intra-uterine device, copper wire, wound on vertical stem of T-shaped plastic carrier with copper sleeves fitted flush on to distal portion of each horizontal arm, total surface area approx. 380 mm², impregnated with barium sulphate for radio-opacity, thread attached to base of vertical stem; easy-loading system, no capsule, net price = £11.70

For minimum uterine length 5 cm; replacement every 5 years (see also notes in BNF section 7.3.4)

Multiload® Cu375

Intra-uterine device, copper wire, surface area approx. 375 mm² vertical stem length 3.5 cm, net price = £9.24

For uterine length 6–9 cm; replacement every 5 years (see also notes in BNF section 7.3.4)

Nova-T® 380

Intra-uterine device, copper wire with silver core, surface area approx. 380 mm² wound on vertical stem of T-shaped plastic carrier, impregnated with barium sulphate for radio-opacity, threads attached to base of vertical stem, net price = £12.97

For uterine length 6.5–9 cm; replacement every 5 years (see also notes in BNF section 7.3.4)

T-Safe® CU 380 A

Intra-uterine device, copper wire, wound on vertical stem of T-shaped plastic carrier with copper collar on the distal portion of each arm, total surface area approx. 380 mm², impregnated with barium sulphate for radio-opacity, threads attached to base of vertical stem, net price = £10.29

For uterine length 6.5–9 cm; replacement every 10 years (see also notes in BNF section 7.3.4)

TT 380 Slimline®

Intra-uterine device, copper wire wound on vertical stem of T-shaped plastic carrier, with copper sleeves fitted flush on to distal portion of each horizontal arm, total surface area approx. 380 mm², impregnated with barium sulphate for

radio-opacity, thread attached to base of vertical stem; easy-loading system, no capsule, net price = £11.70

For uterine length 6.5–9 cm; replacement every 10 years (see also notes in BNF section 7.3.4)

UT 380 Short®

Intra-uterine device, copper wire wound on vertical stem of T-shaped plastic carrier, total surface area approx. 380 mm², impregnated with barium sulphate for radio-opacity, thread attached to base of vertical stem; net price = £10.53

For uterine length 5–7 cm; replacement every 5 years (see also notes in BNF section 7.3.4)

UT 380 Standard®

Intra-uterine device, copper wire, surface area approx. 380 mm², wound on vertical stem of T-shaped plastic carrier, impregnated with barium sulphate for radio-opacity, thread attached to base of vertical stem; net price = £10.53

For uterine length over 5.5–9 cm; replacement every 5 years (see also notes in BNF section 7.3.4)

Other contraceptive devices

◢*Contraceptive caps, prescribe as:*

Soft Silicone cap

Silicone, sizes 22 mm, 26 mm, and 30 mm, net price = £15.29. *Proprietary product: FemCap*

Type A contraceptive cap (pessary)

Opaque rubber, sizes 1 (50 mm), 2 (55 mm), 3 (60 mm), 4 (65 mm), 5 (75 mm), net price = £7.06. *Proprietary product: Dumas Vault Cap*

Type B contraceptive cap (pessary)

Opaque rubber, sizes 22 to 31 mm (rising in steps of 3 mm), net price = £8.34. *Proprietary product: Prentif Cavity Rim Cervical Cap*

Type C contraceptive cap (pessary)

Opaque rubber, sizes 1 to 3 (42, 48 and 54 mm), net price = £7.06. *Proprietary product: Vimule Cap*

◢*Contraceptive diaphragms, prescribe as:*

Reflexions Flat Spring Diaphragm

Transparent rubber with flat metal spring, sizes 55–95 mm (rising in steps of 5 mm), net price = £6.12. *Proprietary product: Reflexions*

Type B Diaphragm with coiled metal rim

Opaque rubber with coiled metal rim, sizes 60–100 mm (rising in steps of 5 mm), net price = £6.79. *Proprietary product: Ortho*

Silicone with coiled metal rim, sizes 60–90 mm (rising in steps of 5 mm), net price = £8.35. *Proprietary product: Milex Omniflex*

Type C Arcing Spring Diaphragm

Opaque rubber with arcing spring, sizes 60–95 mm (rising in steps of 5 mm), net price = £7.49. *Proprietary product: Ortho All-Flex*

Silicone with arcing spring, sizes 60–90 mm (rising in steps of 5 mm), net price = £8.35. *Proprietary product: Milex Arcing Style*

Spermicidal contraceptives

Corresponds to BNF section 7.3.3

Spermicidal contraceptives are useful additional safeguards but do **not** give adequate protection if used alone except where fertility is already significantly diminished. They have two components: a spermicide and a vehicle which itself may have some inhibiting effect on sperm activity. Spermicidal contraceptives are suitable for use with barrier methods, such as diaphragms or caps; however they are not generally recommended for use with condoms, as there is no evidence of any additional protection compared with non-spermicidal lubricants.

Spermicidal contraceptives are not suitable for use in those with or at high risk of sexually transmitted diseases (including HIV); high frequency use of the spermicide nonoxinol '9' has been associated with genital lesions, which may increase the risk of acquiring these infections.

> Products such as petroleum jelly (*Vaseline*), baby oil and oil-based vaginal and rectal preparations are likely to damage condoms and contraceptive diaphragms made from latex rubber, and may render them less effective as a barrier method of contraception and as a protection from sexually transmitted diseases (including HIV).

Gygel®
Gel, nonoxinol '9' 2%, net price 30 g = £4.25
Excipients include hydroxybenzoates (parabens), propylene glycol, sorbic acid
Condoms no evidence of harm to latex condoms and diaphragms

A8 Wound management products and elasticated garments

The information in this appendix corresponds to Appendix 8 of BNF 58 (September 2009).

Products described as **NHS** in this appendix are not in the Drug Tariff, or in the Nurse Prescribers' List.

Wound dressings The correct dressing for wound management depends not only on the type of wound but also on the stage of the healing process. The principal stages of healing are:

- cleansing, removal of debris;
- granulation, vascularisation;
- epithelialisation.

The ideal dressing for moist wound healing needs to ensure that the wound remains:

- moist with exudate, but not macerated;
- free of clinical infection and excessive slough;
- free of toxic chemicals, particles or fibres;
- at the optimum temperature for healing;
- undisturbed by the need for frequent changes;
- at the optimum pH value.

As wound healing passes through its different stages, different types of dressings may be required to satisfy better one or other of these requirements. Under normal circumstances, a moist environment is a necessary part of the wound healing process; exudate provides a moist environment and promotes healing, but excessive exudate can cause maceration of the wound and surrounding healthy tissue. The volume and viscosity of exudate changes as the wound heals. There are certain circumstances where moist wound healing is not appropriate (e.g. gangrenous toes associated with vascular disease).

Advanced wound dressings, (section A8.2) are designed to control the environment for wound healing, for example to donate fluid (**hydrogels**), maintain hydration (**hydrocolloids**), or to absorb wound exudate (**alginates, foams**).

Practices such as the use of irritant cleansers and desloughing agents may be harmful and are largely obsolete; removal of debris and dressing remnants should need minimal irrigation with physiological saline.

Hydrogel, hydrocolloid, and medical grade honey dressings can be used to deslough wounds by promoting autolytic debridement; there is insufficient evidence to support any particular method of debridement for difficult-to-heal surgical wounds. Sterile larvae (maggots) are also available for biosurgical removal of wound debris.

There have been few clinical trials able to establish a clear advantage for any particular product. The choice between different dressings depends not only on the type and stage of the wound, but also on patient preference or tolerance, site of the wound, and cost. For further information, see *Buyers' Guide: Advanced wound dressings* (October 2008); NHS Purchasing and Supply Agency, Centre for Evidence-based Purchasing.

The table below gives suggestions for choices of primary dressing depending on the type of wound (a secondary dressing may be needed in some cases).

A8.1 Basic wound contact dressings

A8.1.1 Low adherence dressings

Low adherence dressings are used as interface layers under secondary absorbent dressings. Placed directly on the wound bed, non-absorbent, low adherence dressings are suitable for clean, granulating, lightly exuding wounds without necrosis, and protect the wound bed from direct contact with secondary dressings. Care must be taken to avoid granulation tissue growing into the weave of these dressings

Tulle dressings are manufactured from cotton or viscose fibres which are impregnated with white or yellow soft paraffin to prevent the fibres from sticking, but this is only partly successful and it may be necessary to change the dressings frequently. The paraffin reduces

Wound contact material for different types of wounds

Wound PINK (Epithelialising)		
Low Exudate	**Moderate Exudate**	
Low adherence A8.1.1 Vapour-permeable film A8.2.2 Soft polymer A.8.2.3 Hydrocolloid A8.2.4	Soft polymer A8.2.3 Foam, low absorbent A8.2.5 Alginate A8.2.6	

Wound RED (Granulating) Symptoms or signs of infection, see **Wounds with signs of infection**		
Low Exudate	**Moderate Exudate**	**Heavy Exudate**
Low adherence A8.1.1 Soft polymer A8.2.3 Hydrocolloid A8.2.4 Foam, low absorbent A8.2.5	Hydrocolloid-fibrous A8.2.4 Foam A8.2.5 Alginate A8.2.6	Foam with extra absorbency A8.2.5 Hydrocolloid-fibrous A8.2.4 Alginate A8.2.6

Wound YELLOW (Sloughy) Symptoms or signs of infection, see **Wounds with signs of infection**		
Low Exudate	**Moderate Exudate**	**Heavy Exudate**
Hydrogel A8.2.1 Hydrocolloid A8.2.4	Hydrocolloid-fibrous A8.2.4 Alginate A8.2.6	Hydrocolloid-fibrous A8.2.4 Alginate A8.2.6 Capillary-action A8.2.7

Wound BLACK (Necrotic/Eschar) Consider mechanical debridement alongside autolytic debridement		
Low Exudate or Dry	**Moderate Exudate**	**Heavy Exudate**
Hydrogel A8.2.1 Hydrocolloid A8.2.4	Hydrocolloid A8.2.4 Hydrocolloid-fibrous A8.2.4 Foam A8.2.5	Seek advice from wound care specialist

Wounds with signs of infection **Consider systemic antibacterials if appropriate;** also consider odour-absorbent dressings (section A8.2.8) For malodourous wounds with slough or necrotic tissue, consider mechanical or autolytic debridement		
Low Exudate	**Moderate Exudate**	**Heavy Exudate**
Low adherence with honey A8.3.1 Low adherence with iodine A8.3.2 Low adherence with silver A8.3.3 Hydrocolloid with silver A8.3.3 Honey—topical A8.3.1	Hydrocolloid-fibrous with silver A8.3.3 Foam with silver A8.3.3 Alginate with silver A8.3.3 Honey—topical A8.3.1 Cadexomer—iodine A8.3.2	Hydrocolloid-fibrous with silver A8.3.3 Foam, extra absorbent, with silver A8.3.3 Alginate with honey A8.3.1 Alginate with silver A8.3.3

Note In each section of this table the dressings are listed in order of increasing absorbency.
Some wound contact (primary) dressings require a secondary dressing

absorbency of the dressing. Dressings with a reduced content of soft paraffin are less liable to interfere with absorption; those containing the traditional amount (such as *Jelonet*®) have been considered more suitable for skin graft transfer.

Knitted viscose primary dressing is an alternative to tulle dressings for exuding wounds; it can be used as the initial layer of multi-layer compression bandaging in the treatment of venous leg ulcers.

Knitted Viscose Primary Dressing, BP 1993
Warp knitted fabric manufactured from a bright viscose monofilament.
N-A Dressing®, 9.5 cm × 9.5 cm = 35p, 9.5 cm × 19 cm = 66p (Systagenix)
N-A Ultra® (silicone-coated), 9.5 cm × 9.5 cm = 33p, 9.5 × 19 cm = 62p (Systagenix)
Paratex®, 9.5 cm × 9.5 cm = 24p (Urgo)
Profore® wound contact layer, 14 cm × 20 cm = 29p (S&N Hlth.)
Tricotex®, 9.5 cm × 9.5 cm = 31p (S&N Hlth.)

Paraffin Gauze Dressing, BP 1993
(Tulle Gras). Fabric of leno weave, weft and warp threads of cotton and/or viscose yarn, impregnated with white or yellow soft paraffin, 10 cm × 10 cm, (light loading) = 25p; (normal loading) = 37p (most suppliers including Synergy Healthcare—*Paranet*® (light loading); BSN Medical—*Cuticell*® *Classic* (normal loading); S&N Hlth.—*Jelonet*® (normal loading); Neomedic—*Neotulle*® (normal loading); C D Medical—*Paragauze*® (normal loading))

Atrauman® (Hartmann)
Non-adherent knitted polyester primary dressing impregnated with neutral triglycerides, 5 cm × 5 cm = 24p, 7.5 cm × 10 cm = 25p, 10 cm × 20 cm = 57p, 20 cm × 30 cm = £1.57

A8.1.2 Absorbent dressings

Perforated film absorbent dressings are suitable only for wounds with mild to moderate amounts of exudate; they are **not** appropriate for leg ulcers or for other lesions that produce large quantities of viscous exudate.

◀For lightly exuding wounds
Absorbent Perforated Dressing with Adhesive Border
Low adherence dressing consisting of viscose and rayon absorbent pad with adhesive border.
Cosmopor E®, 5 cm × 7.2 cm = 7p, 8 cm × 10 cm = 16p, 8 cm × 15 cm = 25p, 10 cm × 20 cm = 41p, 10 cm × 25 cm = 51p, 10 cm × 35 cm = 71p (Hartmann)
Leukomed®, 7.2 cm × 5 cm = 8p, 8 cm × 10 cm = 17p, 8 cm × 15 cm = 30p, 10 cm × 20 cm = 40p, 10 cm × 25 cm = 45p, 10 cm × 30 cm = 58p , 10 cm × 35 cm = 67p (BSN Medical)
Medipore® + Pad, 5 cm × 7.2 cm = 7p, 10 cm × 10 cm = 15p, 10 cm × 15 cm = 24p, 10 cm × 20 cm = 36p, 10 cm × 25 cm = 45p, 10 cm × 35 cm = 62p (3M)
Medisafe®, 6 cm × 8 cm = 8p, 8 cm × 10 cm = 13p, 8 cm × 12 cm = 23p, 9 cm × 15 cm = 29p, 9 cm × 20 cm = 34p, 9 cm × 25 cm = 36p (Neomedic)
Mepore®, 7 cm × 8 cm = 10p, 10 cm × 11 cm = 20p, 11 cm × 15 cm = 34p, 9 cm × 20 cm = 41p, 9 cm × 25 cm = 57p, 9 cm × 30 cm = 65p, 9 cm × 35 cm = 71p (Mölnlycke)
PremierPore®, 5 cm × 7 cm = 5p, 10 cm × 10 cm = 12p, 10 cm × 15 cm = 18p, 10 cm × 20 cm = 32p, 10 cm × 25 cm = 36p, 10 cm × 30 cm = 45p, 10 cm × 35 cm = 52p (Shermond)
Primapore®, 6 cm × 8.3 cm = 16p, 8 cm × 10 cm = 18p, 8 cm × 15 cm = 30p, 10 cm × 20 cm = 40p, 10 cm × 25 cm = 46p, 10 cm × 30 cm = 57p, 10 cm × 35 cm = 88p (S&N Hlth)

Softpore®, 6 cm × 7 cm = 6p, 10 cm × 10 cm = 13p, 10 cm × 15 cm = 20p, 10 cm × 20 cm = 35p, 10 cm × 25 cm = 40p, 10 cm × 30 cm = 49p, 10 cm × 35 cm = 58p (Richardson)
Sterifix®, 5 cm × 7 cm = 18p, 7 cm × 10 cm = 30p, 10 cm × 14 cm = 53p (Hartmann)
Telfa® Island, 5 cm × 10 cm = 8p, 10 cm × 12.5 cm = 27p, 10 cm × 20 cm = 35p, 10 cm × 25.5 cm = 44p, 10 cm × 35 cm = 61p (Covidien)

Absorbent Perforated Plastic Film Faced Dressing
Low-adherence dressing consisting of 3 layers. Where no size specified by the prescriber, the 5 cm size to be supplied
Askina® Pad, 5 cm × 5 cm = 13p, 10 cm × 10 cm = 20p, 10 cm × 20 cm = 40p (Braun)
Cutisorb® LA, 5 cm × 5 cm = 8p, 10 cm × 10 cm = 14p, 10 cm × 20 cm = 29p (BSN Medical)
Interpose®, 5 cm × 5 cm = 9p, 10 cm × 10 cm = 15p, 10 cm × 20 cm = 32p (Frontier)
Melolin®, 5 cm × 5 cm = 16p, 10 cm × 10 cm = 25p, 20 cm × 10 cm = 49p (S&N Hlth)
Release®, 5 cm × 5 cm = 14p, 10 cm × 10 cm = 23p, 20 cm × 10 cm = 43p (Systagenix)
Skintact®, 5 cm × 5 cm = 10p, 10 cm × 10 cm = 17p, 20 cm × 10 cm = 34p (Robinson)
Solvaline N®, 5 cm × 5 cm = 9p, 10 cm × 10 cm = 16p, 10 cm × 20 cm = 33p (Activa)
Telfa®, 5 cm × 7.5 cm = 12p, 10 cm × 7.5 cm = 15p, 15 cm × 7.5 cm = 17p, 20 cm × 7.5 cm = 29p (Covidien)

◀For moderately to heavily exuding wounds
Absorbent Cellulose Dressing with Fluid Repellent Backing
Eclypse®, 15 cm × 15 cm = 97p, 20 cm × 30 cm = £2.14, 60 cm × 40 cm = £8.15, 80 cm × 50 cm = £9.35 (Advancis)
Exu-Dry®, 10 cm × 15 cm = £1.03, 15 cm × 23 cm = £2.11, 23 cm × 38 cm = £4.90 (S&N Hlth.)
Mesorb®, cellulose wadding pad with gauze wound contact layer and non-woven repellent backing, 10 cm × 10 cm = 58p, 10 cm × 15 cm = 75p, 10 cm × 20 cm = 93p, 15 cm × 20 cm = £1.32, 20 cm × 25 cm = £2.08, 20 cm × 30 cm = £2.36 (Mölnlycke)
Telfa Max®, 22.8 cm × 38 cm = £4.62, 38 cm × 45.7 cm = £5.61, 38 cm × 60.9 cm = £8.16 (Covidien)
Zetuvit® E, *non-sterile*, 10 cm × 10 cm = 6p, 10 cm × 20 cm = 8p, 20 cm × 20 cm = 13p, 20 cm × 40 cm = 25p; *sterile*, 10 cm × 10 cm = 19p, 10 cm × 20 cm = 22p, 20 cm × 20 cm = 35p, 20 cm × 40 cm = 98p (Hartmann)

KerraMax® (Ark Therapeutics)
Super absorbent polyacrylate primary dressing, 10 cm × 22 cm = £1.02, 20 cm × 22 cm = £1.80

A8.2 Advanced wound dressings

Advanced wound dressings can be used for both acute and chronic wounds. Categories for dressings in this section (A8.2) start with the least absorptive, moisture-donating hydrogel dressings, followed by increasingly more absorptive dressings. These dressings are classified according to their primary component; some dressings are comprised of several components

A8.2.1 Hydrogel dressings

Hydrogel dressings are most commonly supplied as an amorphous, cohesive topical application that can take up the shape of a wound. A secondary, non-absorbent dressing is needed. These dressings are generally used to donate liquid to dry sloughy wounds and facilitate autolytic debridement of necrotic tissue; some also have the ability to absorb very small amounts of exudate. Hydrogel products that do not contain propylene glycol should be used if the wound is to be treated with larval therapy.

Hydrogel sheets have a fixed structure and limited fluid-handling capacity; hydrogel sheet dressings are best avoided in the presence of infection, and are unsuitable for heavily exuding wounds

◢ Hydrogel sheet dressings
ActiFormCool® (Activa)
Hydrogel dressing, 5 cm × 6.5 cm = £1.65, 10 cm × 10 cm = £2.43, 20 cm × 20 cm = £7.45, 10 cm × 15 cm = £3.49

Aquaflo® (Covidien)
Hydrogel dressing, 7.5 cm diameter = £2.55, 12 cm diameter = £5.26

Coolie® (Zeroderma)
Hydrogel dressing with lint backing, 7 cm diameter = £1.96

Gel FX® (Synergy Healthcare)
Hydrogel dressing (without adhesive border) 10 cm × 10 cm = £1.60, 15 cm × 15 cm = £3.20

Geliperm® (Geistlich)
Hydrogel sheets, 10 cm × 10 cm = £2.27

Hydrosorb® (Hartmann)
Absorbent, transparent, hydrogel sheets containing poly-urethane polymers covered with a semi-permeable film, 5 cm × 7.5 cm = £1.43; 10 cm × 10 cm = £2.04; 20 cm × 20 cm = £6.12
Hydrosorb® comfort (with adhesive border, waterproof), 4.5 cm × 6.5 cm = £1.69; 7.5 cm × 10 cm = £2.24; 12.5 cm × 12.5 cm = £3.26

Intrasite Conformable® (S&N Hlth.)
Soft non-woven dressing impregnated with *Intrasite®* gel, 10 cm × 10 cm = £1.66; 10 cm × 20 cm = £2.23; 10 cm × 40 cm = £3.99

Novogel® (Ford)
Glycerol-based hydrogel sheets, 10 cm × 10 cm = £3.07; 30 cm × 30 cm, standard = £13.00, thin = £12.27; 5 cm × 7.5 cm = £1.95; 15 cm × 20 cm = £5.86; 20 cm × 40 cm = £11.16; 7.5 cm diameter = £2.79

Vacunet® (Protex)
Non-adherent, hydrogel coated polyester net dressing, 10 cm × 10 cm = £1.93, 10 cm × 15 cm = £2.86

◢ Hydrogel application (amorphous)
ActivHeal® Hydrogel (MedLogic)
Hydrogel containing guar gum and propylene glycol, 15 g = £1.36

Aquaform® (Unomedical)
Hydrogel containing modified starch copolymer, 8 g = £1.57, 15 g = £1.91

Askina® Gel (Braun)
Hydrogel containing modified starch and glycerol, 15 g = £1.89

Cutimed® (BSN Medical)
Hydrogel, 8 g = £1.56, 15 g = £1.90, 25 g = £2.80

Flexigran® (A1 Pharmaceuticals)
Hydrogel containing starch polymer and glycerol, 15 g = £1.90

GranuGel® (ConvaTec)
Hydrogel containing carboxymethylcellulose, pectin, and propylene glycol, 15 g = £2.13

Intrasite® Gel (S&N Hlth.)
Hydrogel containing modified carmellose polymer and pro-pylene glycol, 8-g sachet = £1.66, 15-g sachet = £2.22, 25-g sachet = £3.29

Nu-Gel® (Systagenix)
Hydrogel containing alginate and propylene glycol, 15 g = £2.05

Purilon® Gel (Coloplast)
Hydrogel containing carboxymethylcellulose and calcium alginate, 8 g = £1.61, 15 g = £2.10

A8.2.2 Vapour-permeable films and membranes

Vapour-permeable films and membranes allow the passage of water vapour and oxygen but are impermeable to water and micro-organisms, and are suitable for lightly exuding wounds. They are highly conformable, provide protection, and a moist healing environment; transparent film dressings permit constant observation of the wound. Water vapour loss can occur at a slower rate than exudate is generated, so that fluid accumulates under the dressing, which can lead to tissue maceration and to wrinkling at the adhesive contact site (with risk of bacterial entry). Newer versions of these dressings have increased moisture vapour permeability. Despite these advances, vapour-permeable films and membranes are unsuitable for infected, large heavily exuding wounds, and chronic leg ulcers.

Vapour-permeable films and membranes are suitable for partial-thickness wounds with minimal exudate, or wounds with eschar. Most commonly, they are used as a secondary dressing over alginates or hydrogels; film dressings can also be used to protect the fragile skin of patients at risk of developing minor skin damage caused by friction or pressure.

Vapour-permeable Adhesive Film Dressing, BP 1993 (Semi-permeable Adhesive Dressing)
Extensible, waterproof, water vapour-permeable poly-urethane film coated with synthetic adhesive mass; transparent. Supplied in single-use pieces.

ActivHeal® Film, 6 cm × 7 cm = 31p, 10 cm × 12.7 cm = 73p, 15 cm × 17.8 cm = £1.78 (MedLogic)

Askina® Derm, 6 cm × 7 cm = 35p, 10 cm × 12 cm = £1.02, 10 cm × 20 cm = £1.94, 15 cm × 20 cm = £2.35, 20 cm × 30 cm = £4.20 (Braun)

Bioclusive®, 10.2 cm × 12.7 cm = £1.51 (Systagenix)

Blisterfilm®, 5 cm × 7.5 cm = 41p, 9 cm × 10 cm = 71p, 10 cm × 12.5 cm = 92p, 14 cm × 15 cm = £1.25 (Covidien)

C-View®, 6 cm × 7 cm = 39p, 10 cm × 12 cm = £1.08, 12 cm × 12 cm = £1.25, 15 cm × 20 cm = £2.47 (Unomedical)

Episil®, 12 cm × 12 cm = £1.10, 12 cm × 35 cm = £2.75, 15 cm × 20 cm = £2.10 (Advancis)

Hydrofilm®, 6 cm × 7 cm = 21p, 6 cm × 9 cm = 51p, 10 cm × 12.5 cm = 39p, 10 cm × 15 cm = 49p, 10 cm × 25 cm = 76p, 12 cm × 25 cm = 80p, 15 cm × 20 cm = 90p, 20 cm × 30 cm = £1.49 (Hartmann)

Hypafix® Transparent, 10 cm × 2 m = £8.15 (BSN Medical)

Leukomed T®, 7.2 cm × 5 cm = 35p, 8 cm × 10 cm = 65p, 10 cm × 12.5 cm = 95p, 11 cm × 14 cm = £1.15, 15 cm × 20 cm = £2.20, 15 cm × 25 cm = £2.35 (BSN Medical)

Mepore® Film, 6 cm × 7 cm = 43p, 10 cm × 12 cm = £1.14, 10 cm × 25 cm = £2.23, 15 cm × 20 cm = £2.83 (Mölnlycke)

OpSite® Flexifix, (non-sterile) 5 cm × 1 m = £3.59, 10 cm × 1 m = £6.05, OpSite® Flexigrid, 6 cm × 7 cm = 36p, 12 cm × 12 cm = £1.04, 15 cm × 20 cm = £2.62, (S&N Hlth)

Polyskin® II, 4 cm × 4 cm = 36p, 5 cm × 7 cm = 39p, 10 cm × 12 cm = £1.01, 10 cm × 20 cm = £2.00, 15 cm × 20 cm = £2.31, 20 cm × 25 cm = £4.03 (Covidien)

ProtectFilm®, 6 cm × 7 cm = 11p, 10 cm × 12 cm = 20p, 15 cm × 20 cm = 40p (Wallace Cameron)

Suprasorb F®, 5 cm × 7 cm = 31p, 10 cm × 12 cm = 73p, 15 cm × 20 cm = £2.30, (Activa)

Tegaderm®, 6 cm × 7 cm = 38p, 12 cm × 12 cm = £1.23, 15 cm × 20 cm = £2.34 (3M)

Vacuskin®, 6 cm × 7 cm = 40p, 10 cm × 12 cm = £1.06, 10 cm × 25 cm = £2.06, 15 cm × 20 cm = £2.19 (Protex)

◢With absorbent pad
Vapour-permeable Adhesive Film Dressing with absorbent pad

Alldress®, with absorbent pad, 10 cm × 10 cm = 88p, 15 cm × 15 cm = £1.92, 15 cm × 20 cm = £2.37 (Mölnlycke)

Hydrofilm® Plus, with absorbent pad, 5 cm × 7.2 cm = 15p, 9 cm × 10 cm = 20p, 9 cm × 15 cm = 22p, 10 cm × 20 cm = 34p, 10 cm × 25 cm = 36p, 10 cm × 30 cm = 53p (Hartmann)

Leukomed T® Plus, with absorbent pad, 7.2 cm × 5 cm = 25p, 8 cm × 10 cm = 50p, 8 cm × 15 cm = 75p, 10 cm × 20 cm = £1.25, 10 cm × 25 cm = £1.40, 10 cm × 30 cm = £2.35, 10 cm × 35 cm = £2.85 (BSN Medical)

Mepore® Ultra, with absorbent pad, 6 cm × 7 cm = 28p, 7 cm × 8 cm = 38p, 9 cm × 10 cm = 61p, 9 cm × 15 cm = 92p, 9 cm × 20 cm = £1.39, 9 cm × 25 cm = £1.54, 9 cm × 30 cm = £2.54, 10 cm × 11 cm = 74p, 11 cm × 15 cm = £1.10 (Mölnlycke)

OpSite® Plus, with absorbent pad, 5 cm × 5 cm = 29p, 9.5 cm × 8.5 cm = 81p, 10 cm × 12 cm = £1.10, 10 cm × 20 cm = £1.85, 35 cm × 10 cm = £3.07 (S&N Hlth)

Pharmapore-PU®, with absorbent pad, 8.5 cm × 15.5 cm = 20p, 10 cm × 25 cm = 38p, 10 cm × 30 cm = 58p (Wallace Cameron)

PremierPore VP®, with absorbent pad, 5 cm × 7 cm = 13p, 6 cm × 7 cm = 21p, 10 cm × 10 cm = 16p, 10 cm × 15 cm = 24p, 10 cm × 20 cm = 36p, 10 cm × 25 cm = 38p, 10 cm × 30 cm = 57p, 10 cm × 35 cm = 69p (Shermond)

Tegaderm®, with absorbent pad, 5 cm × 7 cm = 25p, 9 cm × 10 cm = 62p, 9 cm × 15 cm = 92p, 9 cm × 20 cm = £1.34, 9 cm × 25 cm = £1.51, 9 cm × 35 cm = £2.50 (3M)

◢For intravenous and subcutaneous catheter sites
Central Gard® (Unomedical)

16 cm × 7 cm (central venous catheter) = 94p, 16 cm × 8.8 cm (central venous catheter) = £1.03

Easl-V® (ConvaTec)

7 cm × 7.5 cm (intravenous peripheral cannula) = 38p

IV3000® (S&N Hlth.)

5 cm × 6 cm (1-hand) = 39p, 6 cm × 7 cm (non-winged peripheral catheter) = 51p, 7 cm × 9 cm (ported peripheral catheter) = 67p, 9 cm × 12 cm (PICC line) = £1.34, 10 cm × 12 cm (central venous catheter) = £1.28

Mepore® IV (Mölnlycke)

5 cm × 5.5 cm = 29p, 8 cm × 9 cm = 37p, 10 cm × 11 cm = 97p

Niko Fix® (Unomedical)

7 cm × 8.5 cm (intravenous ported peripheral catheter) = 19p

Pharmapore-PU® IV (Wallace Cameron)

8.5 cm × 7 cm (ported peripheral cannula) = 7p, 6 cm × 7 cm (ported peripheral cannula) = 8p, 7 cm × 9 cm (peripheral cannula, hand) = 17p

Tegaderm® IV (3M)

7 cm × 8.5 cm (peripheral catheter) = 57p, 8.5 cm × 10.5 cm (central venous catheter) = £1.11, 10 cm × 15.5 cm (peripherally inserted central venous catheter) = £1.60

A8.2.3 Soft polymer dressings

Dressings with soft polymer, often a soft silicone polymer, in a non-adherent layer are suitable for use on lightly to moderately exuding wounds. For moderately to heavily exuding wounds, an absorbent secondary dressing can be added, or a soft polymer dressing with an absorbent pad can be used.

Wound contact dressings coated with soft silicone have gentle adhesive properties and can be used on fragile skin areas or where it is beneficial to reduce the frequency of primary dressing changes.

Soft polymer dressings should not be used on heavily bleeding wounds; blood clots can cause the dressing to adhere to the wound surface.

For *silicone keloid dressings* see section A8.4.2.

Mepitel® (Mölnlycke)

Soft silicone wound contact dressing. 5 cm × 7 cm = £1.52, 8 cm × 10 cm = £3.05, 12 cm × 15 cm = £6.17, 20 cm × 30 cm = £16.61

Physiotulle® (Coloplast)

Non-adherent soft polymer wound contact dressing, 10 cm × 10 cm = £2.09, 15 cm × 20 cm = £6.37

Silon-TSR® (Jobskin)

Soft silicone polymer wound contact dressing, 13 cm × 13 cm = £3.52, 13 cm × 25 cm = £5.47, 28 cm × 30 cm = £7.37

Siltex® (Advancis)

Soft silicone-coated polyester wound contact dressing, 5 cm × 7 cm = £1.25, 8 cm × 10 cm = £2.55, 12 cm × 15 cm = £5.15, 20 cm × 30 cm = £13.25

Tegaderm® Contact (3M)

Non-adherent soft polymer wound contact dressing, 7.5 cm × 10 cm = £2.14, 7.5 cm × 20 cm = £4.20, 20 cm × 25 cm = £10.23

Urgotul® (Urgo)

Non-adherent soft polymer wound contact dressing, 11 cm × 11 cm = £3.00, 10 cm × 40 cm = £9.89, 16 cm × 21 cm = £8.49

Urgotul® Start, soft polymer wound contact dressing, 5 cm × 7 cm = £2.80, 11 cm × 11 cm = £3.98, 16 cm × 21 cm = £9.50

◢With absorbent pad
Allevyn® Gentle (S&N Hlth.)

Soft gel wound contact dressing, with polyurethane foam film backing, 5 cm × 5 cm = £1.23, 10 cm × 10 cm = £2.43, 10 cm × 20 cm = £3.91, 15 cm × 15 cm = £4.40, 20 cm × 20 cm = £6.52

Allevyn® Gentle Border, silicone gel wound contact dressing, with polyurethane foam film backing, 7.5 cm × 7.5 cm = £1.43, 10 cm × 10 cm = £2.44, 12.5 cm × 12.5 cm = £3.14, 17.5 cm × 17.5 cm = £6.11, 23 cm × 23.2 cm (heel) = £8.95

Eclypse® Adherent (Advancis)

Soft silicone wound contact layer with absorbent pad and film-backing, 10 cm × 10 cm = £2.99, 10 cm × 20 cm = £3.75, 15 cm × 15 cm = £4.99, 20 cm × 30 cm = £9.99

Episil® Absorbent (Advancis)

Soft silicone wound contact dressing, with polyurethane foam film backing, 7.5 cm × 7.5 cm = £1.19, 10 cm × 10 cm = £2.16, 10 cm × 20 cm = £2.90, 10 cm × 30 cm = £4.25, 15 cm × 15 cm = £3.15, 15 cm × 20 cm = £4.10

Flivasorb® (Activa)

Absorbent polymer dressing with non-adherent wound contact layer, 10 cm × 10 cm = £2.09, 20 cm × 20 cm = £6.58, 10 cm × 20 cm = £3.50

Mepilex® (Mölnlycke)

Absorbent soft silicone dressing with polyurethane foam film backing, 10 cm × 11 cm = £2.53, 11 cm × 20 cm = £4.18, 15 cm × 16 cm = £4.59, 20 cm × 21 cm = £6.93, 20 cm × 50 cm = £27.24

Mepilex® Border, absorbent soft silicone dressing with polyurethane foam and adhesive border, 7 cm × 7.5 cm = £1.31, 10 cm × 12.5 cm = £2.59, 10 cm × 20 cm = £3.47, 10 cm × 30 cm = £5.21, 15 cm × 17.5 cm = £4.46, 17 cm × 20 cm = £5.78

Mepilex® Border Lite, thin absorbent soft silicone dressing with polyurethane foam and adhesive border, 4 cm × 5 cm = 88p, 7.5 cm × 7.5 cm = £1.33, 5 cm × 12.5 cm = £1.92, 10 cm × 10 cm = £2.42, 15 cm × 15 cm = £3.95; 18 cm × 18 cm (sacrum) = £4.56, 23 cm × 23 cm (sacrum) = £7.44; 13 cm × 20 cm (heel) = £5.15

Mepilex® Lite, thin absorbent soft silicone dressing with polyurethane foam, 6 cm × 8.5 cm = £1.69, 10 cm × 10 cm = £2.02, 15 cm × 15 cm = £3.92, 20 cm × 50 cm = £24.77

Mepilex® Transfer, soft silicone exudate transfer dressing, 7.5 cm × 8.5 cm = £2.10, 10 cm × 12 cm = £3.30, 15 cm × 20 cm = £9.89, 20 cm × 50 cm = £25.27

Proguide® (S&N Hlth.)

Non-adherent polyurethane wound contact layer with absorbent pad, 10 cm × 10 cm = £2.00

Sorbion® Sana (H&R)

Non-adherent polyethylene wound contact layer with absorbent core, 8.5 cm × 8.5 cm = £4.93, 12 cm × 12 cm = £6.68, 12 cm × 22 cm = £12.37, 22 cm × 22 cm = £19.84

UrgoCell® (Urgo)

Non-adherent soft polymer wound contact dressing with polyurethane foam film backing, 10 cm × 12 cm = £4.44, 15 cm × 20 cm = £9.00; with adhesive border 13 cm × 13 cm = £4.44, 15 cm × 20 cm = £9.00

UrgoCell Start®, soft polymer wound contact dressing with polyurethane foam backing, 6 cm × 6 cm = £4.30, 10 cm × 10 cm = £5.95, 15 cm × 20 cm = £10.70

Urgotul® Duo (Urgo)

Non-adherent, soft polymer wound contact dressing with absorbent pad, 5 cm × 10 cm = £2.29, 10 cm × 12 cm = £3.54, 15 cm × 20 cm = £8.22

Urgotul® Duo Border, soft polymer wound contact dressing with absorbent pad and adhesive polyurethane film backing, 8 cm × 8 cm = £2.24, 10 cm × 12 cm = £3.47, 15 cm × 20 cm = £8.05

◀ **Bio-cellulose dressings**

Suprasorb® X (Activa)

Biosynthetic cellulose fibre dressing, 5 cm × 5 cm = £1.87, 9 cm × 9 cm = £3.89, 14 cm × 20 cm = £7.71; 2 cm × 21 cm (rope) = £5.99

A8.2.4 Hydrocolloid dressings

Hydrocolloid dressings are usually presented as a hydrocolloid layer on a vapour-permeable film or foam pad. Semi-permeable to water vapour and oxygen, these dressings form a gel in the presence of exudate to facilitate rehydration in lightly to moderately exuding wounds and promote autolytic debridement of dry, sloughy, or necrotic wounds; they are also suitable for promoting granulation.

Hydrocolloid-fibrous dressings made from modified carmellose fibres resemble alginate dressings; hydrocolloid-fibrous dressings are more absorptive and suitable for moderately to heavily exuding wounds.

◀ **Without adhesive border**

ActivHeal® Hydrocolloid (MedLogic)

Semi-permeable polyurethane film backing, hydrocolloid wound contact layer, 5 cm × 7.5 cm = 75p, 10 cm × 10 cm =

£1.52, 15 cm × 15 cm = £3.31, 15 cm × 18 cm (sacral) = £3.84; with polyurethane foam layer, 5 cm × 7.5 cm = 94p, 10 cm × 10 cm = £1.49, 15 cm × 15 cm = £2.81, 15 cm × 18 cm (sacral) = £3.24

Alione® (Coloplast)

Semi-permeable hydrocolloid dressing without adhesive border, 10 cm × 10 cm = £2.96, 12.5 cm × 12.5 cm = £4.07, 12 cm × 20 cm = £5.34, 15 cm × 15 cm = £5.14, 20 cm × 20 cm = £7.68

Askina® Biofilm Transparent (Braun)

Semi-permeable, polyurethane film dressing with hydrocolloid adhesive, 10 cm × 10 cm = £1.02, 15 cm × 15 cm = £2.31, 20 cm × 20 cm = £3.02

Comfeel® Plus (Coloplast)

Hydrocolloid dressings containing carmellose sodium and calcium alginate. contour, 6 cm × 8 cm = £2.04, 9 cm × 11 cm = £3.54; ulcer, 4 cm × 6 cm = 88p, 10 cm × 10 cm = £2.25, 15 cm × 15 cm = £4.82, 18 cm × 20 cm (triangular) = £5.25, 20 cm × 20 cm = £6.94; transparent, 5 cm × 7 cm = 61p, 5 cm × 15 cm = £1.46, 5 cm × 25 cm = £2.37, 9 cm × 14 cm = £2.24, 9 cm × 25 cm = £3.18, 10 cm × 10 cm = £1.17, 15 cm × 15 cm = £3.06, 15 cm × 20 cm = £3.11, 17 cm × 14 cm (sacral) = £3.44, 20 cm × 20 cm = £3.13; pressure relieving, 7 cm diameter = £3.18, 10 cm = £4.26, 15 cm = £6.42

DuoDERM® Extra Thin (ConvaTec)

Semi-permeable hydrocolloid dressing, 5 cm × 10 cm = 71p, 7.5 cm × 7.5 cm = 73p, 10 cm × 10 cm = £1.21, 9 cm × 15 cm = £1.63, 9 cm × 25 cm = £2.61, 9 cm × 35 cm = £3.65, 15 cm × 15 cm = £2.61

DuoDERM® Signal, hydrocolloid dressing with 'Time to change' indicator, 10 cm × 10 cm = £1.97, 14 cm × 14 cm = £3.45, 20 cm × 20 cm = £6.86, 11 cm × 19 cm (oval) = £2.99, 18.5 cm × 19.5 cm (heel) = £4.82, 22.5 cm × 20 cm (sacral) = £5.64

Flexigran® (A1 Pharmaceuticals)

Semi-permeable hydrocolloid dressing without adhesive border, 10 cm × 10 cm = £2.19; thin, 10 cm × 10 cm = £1.08

Granuflex® (ConvaTec)

Hydrocolloid wound contact layer bonded to plastic foam layer, with outer semi-permeable polyurethane film, 10 cm × 10 cm = £2.56, 15 cm × 15 cm = £4.87, 15 cm × 20 cm = £5.27, 20 cm × 20 cm = £7.32

Hydrocoll® Basic (Hartmann)

Hydrocolloid dressing with absorbent wound contact pad, 10 cm × 10 cm = £2.23; thin, 7.5 cm × 7.5 cm = 63p, 10 cm × 10 cm = £1.05, 15 cm × 15 cm = £2.36

NU DERM® (Systagenix)

Semi-permeable hydrocolloid dressing, 5 cm × 5 cm = 83p, 10 cm × 10 cm = £1.53, 15 cm × 15 cm = £3.12, 20 cm × 20 cm = £6.24, 8 cm × 12 cm (heel/elbow) = £3.12, 15 cm × 18 cm (sacral) = £4.37; thin, 10 cm × 10 cm = £1.04

Suprasorb® H (Activa)

Semi-permeable hydrocolloid dressing, without adhesive border 10 cm × 10 cm = £1.54, 15 cm × 15 cm = £3.37; thin, 5 cm × 10 cm = 66p, 10 cm × 10 cm = £1.01, 15 cm × 15 cm = £2.31

Tegaderm® Hydrocolloid (3M)

Hydrocolloid dressing without adhesive border, 10 cm × 10 cm = £2.30, 15 cm × 15 cm = £4.46; thin, semi-permeable, clear film dressing with hydrocolloid, 10 cm × 10 cm = £1.51

Ultec Pro® (Covidien)

Semi-permeable hydrocolloid dressing; without adhesive border 10 cm × 10 cm = £2.23, 15 cm × 15 cm = £4.36, 20 cm × 20 cm = £6.56

◀ **With adhesive border**

Alione® (Coloplast)

Semi-permeable hydrocolloid dressing with adhesive border, 10 cm × 10 cm = £2.96, 12.5 cm × 12.5 cm = £4.07, 12 cm × 20 cm = £5.34, 15 cm × 15 cm = £5.14, 20 cm × 20 cm = £7.68

Granulflex® Bordered (ConvaTec)

Hydrocolloid wound contact layer bonded to plastic foam layer, with outer semi-permeable polyurethane film, 6 cm × 6 cm = £1.63, 10 cm × 10 cm = £3.06, 15 cm × 15 cm = £5.88, 10 cm × 13 cm (triangular) = £3.61, 15 cm × 18 cm (triangular) = £5.62

Hydrocoll® Border (Hartmann)

Hydrocolloid dressing with adhesive border and absorbent wound contact pad, 5 cm × 5 cm = 92p, 7.5 cm × 7.5 cm = £1.51, 10 cm × 10 cm = £2.20, 15 cm × 15 cm = £4.13; 8 cm × 12 cm (concave) = £1.93; 12 cm × 18 cm (sacral) = £3.29

Suprasorb® H (Activa)

Semi-permeable hydrocolloid dressing with adhesive border, 14 cm × 14 cm = £2.27

Tegaderm® Hydrocolloid (3M)

Hydrocolloid dressing with adhesive border, 10 cm × 12 cm (oval) = £2.26, 13 cm × 15 cm (oval) = £4.22; 17.1 cm × 16.1 cm (sacral) = £4.71; *thin*, semi-permeable, clear film dressing with hydrocolloid 10 cm × 12 cm (oval) = £1.50; 13 cm × 15 cm (oval) = £2.81

Ultec Pro® (Covidien)

Semi-permeable hydrocolloid dressing with adhesive border, 21 cm × 21 cm = £4.58, 15 cm × 18 cm (sacral) = £3.23, 19.5 cm × 23 cm (sacral) = £4.88

◢**Hydrocolloid-fibrous dressings**

Aquacel® (ConvaTec)

Soft non-woven pad containing hydrocolloid-fibres, 4 cm × 10 cm = £1.38, 4 cm × 20 cm = £2.04, 4 cm × 30 cm = £3.05, 5 cm × 5 cm = £1.07; 10 cm × 10 cm = £2.54; 15 cm × 15 cm = £4.78; 2 cm × 45 cm (ribbon) = £2.59

Versiva® XC (ConvaTec)

Hydrocolloid gelling foam dressing, without adhesive border, 7.5 cm × 7.5 cm = £1.35, 11 cm × 11 cm = £2.25, 15 cm × 15 cm = £4.15, 20 cm × 20 cm = £6.20; with adhesive border, 10 cm × 10 cm = £2.30, 14 cm × 14 cm = £3.10, 19 cm × 19 cm = £4.95, 22 cm × 22 cm = £5.50, 18.5 cm × 20.5 cm (heel) = £5.50, 21 cm × 25 cm (sacral) = £5.90

◢**Polyurethane matrix dressing**

Cutinova® Hydro (S&N Hlth.)

Polyurethane matrix with absorbent particles and waterproof polyurethane film, 5 cm × 6 cm = £1.16, 10 cm × 10 cm = £2.33, 15 cm × 20 cm = £4.94

A8.2.5 Foam dressings

Dressings containing hydrophilic polyurethane foam (adhesive or non-adhesive), with or without plastic film-backing, are suitable for all types of exuding wounds, but not for dry wounds; some foam dressings have a moisture-sensitive film backing with variable permeability dependant on the level of exudate

Foam dressings vary in their ability to absorb exudate; some are suitable only for lightly to moderately exuding wounds, others have greater fluid-handing capacity and are suitable for heavily exuding wounds. Saturated foam dressings can cause maceration of healthy skin if left in contact with the wound.

Foam dressings can be used in combination with other primary wound contact dressings. If used under compression bandaging or compression garments, the fluid-handling capacity of the foam dressing may be reduced. Foam dressings can also be used to provide a protective cushion for fragile skin.

◢**For lightly exuding wounds**

Polyurethane Foam Film Dressing with Adhesive Border

PolyMem®, 5 cm × 5 cm = 48p (Unomedical)

Tielle® Lite, 11 cm × 11 cm = £2.24; 7 cm × 9 cm = £1.19; 8 cm × 15 cm = £2.76; 8 cm × 20 cm = £2.91 (Systagenix)

◢**For lightly to moderately exuding wounds**

Polyurethane Foam Dressing, BP 1993

Lyofoam®, 7.5 cm × 7.5 cm = £1.02, 10 cm × 10 cm = £1.17, 10 cm × 17.5 cm = £1.88, 15 cm × 20 cm = £2.54

Suprasorb® M, 10 cm × 10 cm = £1.75, 10 cm × 20 cm = £3.09, 20 cm × 20 cm = £5.15 (Activa)

Polyurethane Foam Film Dressing with Adhesive Border

Suprasorb® P, 7.5 cm × 7.5 cm = £1.18, 10 cm × 10 cm = £1.28, 15 cm × 15 cm = £2.28 (Activa)

Tielle®, 11 cm × 11 cm = £2.33; 15 cm × 15 cm = £3.81, 18 cm × 18 cm = £4.85, 7 cm × 9 cm = £1.25, 15 cm × 20 cm = £4.77, 18 cm × 18 cm (sacral) = £3.53 (Systagenix)

Polyurethane Foam Film Dressing without Adhesive Border

ActivHeal FlexiPore®, self-adhesive, 6 cm × 7 cm = 93p; 10 cm × 10 cm = £1.73, 15 cm × 20 cm = £3.70; 20 cm × 20 cm = £5.06; 10 cm × 30 cm = £3.60 (MedLogic)

Allevyn® Lite, 5 cm × 5 cm = £1.04; 10 cm × 10 cm = £1.88; 10 cm × 20 cm = £3.22; 15 cm × 20 cm = £4.02 (S&N Hlth.)

Allevyn® Thin, self-adhesive, 5 cm × 6 cm = 98p, 10 cm × 10 cm = £1.98, 15 cm × 15 cm = £3.26, 15 cm × 20 cm = £3.96 (S&N Hlth)

Suprasorb® P, 5 cm × 5 cm = 92p, 7.5 cm × 7.5 cm = 98p, 10 cm × 10 cm = £1.15, 15 cm × 15 cm = £3.07 (Activa)

Transorbent®, self-adhesive, 5 cm × 7 cm = £1.00; 10 cm × 10 cm = £1.89; 15 cm × 15 cm = £3.47; 20 cm × 20 cm = £5.55 (Unomedical)

◢**For moderately to heavily exuding wounds**

Polyurethane Foam Dressing

Copa®, 5 cm × 5 cm = 70p, 7.5 cm × 7.5 cm = £1.19, 10 cm × 10 cm = £1.04, 12.5 cm × 12.5 cm = £1.77, 15 cm × 15 cm = £2.55, 20 cm × 20 cm = £2.95, 10 cm × 20 cm = £2.01, 8.5 cm × 7.5 cm (fenestrated) = 89p (Covidien)

Polyurethane Foam Film Dressing with Adhesive Border

ActivHeal® Foam Island, 10 cm × 10 cm = £1.57, 12.5 cm × 12.5 cm = £1.50, 15 cm × 15 cm = £1.92, 20 cm × 20 cm = £4.34 (MedLogic)

Avazorb® Border, 6 cm × 10 cm = £1.10, 8 cm × 12 cm = £1.90 (Advancis)

Allevyn® Adhesive, 7.5 cm × 7.5 cm = £1.39, 10 cm × 10 cm = £2.00, 12.5 cm × 12.5 cm = £2.50, 17.5 cm × 17.5 cm = £4.93, 12.5 cm × 22.5 cm = £3.89, 22.5 cm × 22.5 cm = £7.18; (sacral) 17 cm x 17 cm = £3.70, 22 cm x 22 cm = £5.32 (S&N Hlth.)

Allevyn® Plus Adhesive, 12.5 cm × 12.5 cm = £3.08; 17.5 cm × 17.5 cm = £5.93; 12.5 cm × 22.5 cm = £5.45; (sacral) 17 cm x 17 cm = £4.48, 22 cm x 22 cm = £6.49 (S&N Hlth)

Biatain® Adhesive, 10 cm × 10 cm = £1.62; 12 cm × 12 cm = £2.38, 18 cm × 18 cm = £4.77, 18 cm × 28 cm = £7.06, 23 cm × 23 cm (sacral) = £4.08, 19 cm × 20 cm (heel) = £4.76; 17 cm diameter (contour) = £4.59 (Coloplast)

Copa® Island, 10 cm × 10 cm = £1.51, 15 cm × 15 cm = £2.84, 20 cm × 20 cm = £5.36 (Coviden)

Lyofoam® Extra Adhesive, 9 cm × 9 cm = £1.27; 15 cm × 15 cm = £2.39; 22 cm × 22 cm = £4.70; 15 cm × 13 cm (sacral) = £1.95 (Medlock)

PermaFoam®, 16.5 cm × 18 cm (concave) = £3.67; 18 cm × 18 cm (sacral) = £3.02; 22 cm × 22 cm (sacral) = £3.47; *PermaFoam Comfort®* 8 cm × 8 cm = £1.02, 10 cm × 20 cm = £3.06, 11 cm × 11 cm = £1.94, 15 cm × 15 cm = £3.16, 20 cm × 20 cm = £4.59 (Hartmann)

PolyMem®, 5 cm × 7.6 cm = £1.07, 8.8 cm × 12.7 cm = £1.90, 10 cm × 13 cm = £2.06, 15 cm × 15 cm = £2.77, 16.5 cm × 20.9 cm = £6.25, 18.4 cm × 20 cm (sacral) = £4.28 (Unomedical)

Tegaderm® Foam Adhesive, 10 cm × 11 cm = £2.30, 14 cm × 14 cm = £3.40, 14 cm × 15 cm = £4.08, 19 cm × 22.5 cm = £6.69, 14 cm × 14 cm (heel) = £4.09 (3M)

Tielle® Plus, 11 cm × 11 cm = £2.58; 15 cm × 15 cm = £4.21; 15 cm × 20 cm = £5.28; 15 cm × 15 cm (sacrum) = £3.07; 20 cm × 26.5 cm (heel) = £4.37 (Systagenix)

Trufoam®, 11 cm × 11 cm = £2.16, 15 cm × 15 cm = £3.62, 7 cm × 9 cm = £1.13, 15 cm × 20 cm = £4.53 (Unomedical)

Polyurethane Foam Film Dressing without Adhesive Border

ActivHeal® Foam Non-Adhesive, 5 cm × 5 cm = 72p, 10 cm × 10 cm = £1.09, 10 cm × 17.8 cm = £2.26, 20 cm × 20 cm = £3.78 (MedLogic)

Advazorb® Plus, 5 cm × 7.5 cm = 70p, 10 cm × 10 cm = £1.08, 15 cm × 15 cm = £2.10, 20 cm × 20 cm = £3.75 (Advancis)

Allevyn®, 5 cm × 5 cm = £1.18, 10 cm × 10 cm = £2.33, 10 cm × 20 cm = £3.75, 20 cm × 20 cm = £6.27, 10.5 cm × 13.5 cm (heel) = £4.68 (S&N Hlth.)

Allevyn® Cavity, circular, 5 cm diameter = £3.86, 10 cm diameter = £9.21; tubular, 9 cm × 2.5 cm = £3.75, 12 cm × 4 cm = £6.60 (S&N Hlth.)

Allevyn® Compression, 5 cm × 6 cm = £1.15; 10 cm × 10 cm = £2.36; 15 cm × 15 cm = £4.01, 15 cm × 20 cm = £4.49 (S&N Hlth.)

Allevyn® Plus Cavity, 5 cm × 6 cm = £1.74, 10 cm × 10 cm = £2.89, 15 cm × 20 cm = £5.79 (S&N Hlth.)

Askina® Foam, 10 cm × 10 cm = £2.06, 10 cm × 20 cm = £3.25, 20 cm × 20 cm = £5.43, 12 cm × 20 cm (heel) = £4.40; cavity dressing, 2.4 cm × 40 cm = £2.30 (Braun)

Biatain® Non-Adhesive, 10 cm × 10 cm = £2.20, 10 cm × 20 cm = £3.63, 15 cm × 15 cm = £4.05, 20 cm × 20 cm = £6.01; 5 cm × 7 cm = £1.21, 5 cm diameter = £1.13, 8 cm diameter = £1.59; Biatain® Soft-Hold, 10 cm × 10 cm = £2.39, 15 cm × 15 cm = £3.97, 5 cm × 7 cm = £1.21, 10 cm × 20 cm = £3.63 (Coloplast)

Copa® Plus, 5 cm × 5 cm = 80p, 7.5 cm × 7.5 cm = £1.39, 10 cm × 10 cm = £1.44, 12.5 cm × 12.5 cm = £2.20, 15 cm × 15 cm = £3.32, 20 cm × 20 cm = £3.96, 10 cm × 20 cm = £2.64, 8.5 cm × 7.5 cm (fenestrated) = £1.22 (Covidien)

Kerraboot®, (clear or white), foot-shaped, extra small = £14.38, small = £14.66, large = £14.66, extra large = £14.38 (Ark)

Lyofoam® Extra, 10 cm × 10 cm = £2.02, 17.5 cm × 10 cm = £3.43, 20 cm × 15 cm = £4.44 (Medlock)

PermaFoam®, 10 cm × 10 cm = £1.94, 10 cm × 20 cm = £3.32, 15 cm × 15 cm = £3.67, 20 cm × 20 cm = £5.61; 6 cm diameter = £1.00, 8 cm × 8 cm (fenestrated) = £1.14; cavity dressing, 10 cm × 10 cm = £1.84 (Hartmann)

PolyMem®, 8 cm × 8 cm = £1.50, 10 cm × 10 cm = £2.34, 13 cm × 13 cm = £3.90, 17 cm × 19 cm = £5.75, 10 cm × 61 cm = £12.39; PolyMem® Max 11 cm × 11 cm = £2.81 (Unomedical)

Tegaderm® Foam, 8.8 cm × 8.8 cm (fenestrated) = £2.14, 10 cm × 10 cm = £2.10, 10 cm × 20 cm = £3.57, 20 cm × 20 cm = £5.69, 10 cm × 60 cm = £12.05 (3M)

Tielle® Plus Borderless, 11 cm × 11 cm = £3.04; 15 cm × 20 cm = £5.51 (Systagenix)

Tielle® Xtra, 11 cm × 11 cm = £2.20; 15 cm × 15 cm = £3.30, 15 cm × 20 cm = £5.40 (Systagenix)

Trufoam® NA, 5 cm × 5 cm = £1.08, 10 cm × 10 cm = £2.05, 15 cm × 15 cm = £3.78 (Unomedical)

Cavi-Care® (S&N Hlth.)

Soft, conforming cavity wound dressing prepared by mixing thoroughly for 15 seconds immediately before use and allowing to expand its volume within the cavity. 20 g = £18.12

A8.2.6 Alginate dressings

Non-woven or fibrous, non-occlusive, alginate dressings, made from calcium alginate, or calcium sodium alginate, derived from brown seaweed, form a soft gel in contact with wound exudate.

Alginate dressings are highly absorbent and suitable for use on exuding wounds, and for the promotion of autolytic debridement of debris in very moist wounds. Alginate dressings also act as a haemostatic, but caution is needed because blood clots can cause the dressing to adhere to the wound surface. Alginate dressings should not be used if bleeding is heavy and extreme caution is needed if used for tumours with friable tissue.

Alginate sheets are suitable for use as a wound contact dressing for moderately to heavily exuding wounds and can be layered into deep wounds; alginate rope can be used in sinus and cavity wounds to improve absorption of exudate and prevent maceration. If the dressing does not have an adhesive border or integral adhesive plastic film backing, a secondary dressing will be required.

ActivHeal® (MedLogic)

Activheal® Alginate, calcium sodium alginate dressing, 5 cm × 5 cm = 57p, 10 cm × 10 cm = £1.11, 10 cm × 20 cm = £2.73; cavity dressing, 2 cm × 30 cm = £2.05

ActivHeal Aquafiber®, non-woven, calcium sodium alginate dressing, 5 cm × 5 cm = 73p, 10 cm × 10 cm = £1.74, 15 cm × 15 cm = £3.28; cavity dressing, 2 cm × 42 cm = £1.75

Algisite® M (S&N Hlth.)

Calcium alginate fibre, non-woven dressing, 5 cm × 5 cm = 85p, 10 cm × 10 cm = £1.75, 15 cm × 20 cm = £4.71; cavity dressing, 2 cm × 30 cm = £3.18

Algosteril® (S&N Hlth.)

Calcium alginate dressing. 5 cm × 5 cm = 84p, 10 cm × 10 cm = £1.92, 10 cm × 20 cm = £3.25; cavity dressing, 2 g, 30 cm = £3.47

Curasorb® (Covidien)

Calcium alginate dressing, 5 cm × 5 cm = 70p, 10 cm × 10 cm = £1.49, 10 cm × 14 cm = £2.41, 10 cm × 20 cm = £2.93, 15 cm × 25 cm = £5.15, 30 cm × 61 cm = £27.03; cavity dressing, 30 cm = £2.84, 61 cm = £4.98, 91 cm = £5.36

Curasorb® Plus, calcium alginate dressing, 10 cm × 10 cm = £2.04

Curasorb® Zn, calcium alginate and zinc dressing, 5 cm × 5 cm = 80p, 10 cm × 10 cm = £1.68, 10 cm × 20 cm = £3.30

Kaltostat® (ConvaTec)

Calcium alginate fibre, non-woven, 5 cm × 5 cm, = 87p, 7.5 cm × 12 cm = £1.91, 10 cm × 20 cm = £3.77, 15 cm × 25 cm = £6.48; cavity dressing, 2 g = £3.54

Melgisorb® (Mölnlycke)

Calcium sodium alginate fibre, highly absorbent, gelling dressing, non-woven, 5 cm × 5 cm = 84p, 10 cm × 10 cm = £1.74, 10 cm × 20 cm = £3.27; cavity dressing, 32 cm × 2.2 cm, (2 g) = £3.30

SeaSorb® (Coloplast)

SeaSorb® Soft, alginate containing hydrocolloid dressing, highly absorbent, gelling dressing, 5 cm × 5 cm = 90p, 10 cm × 10 cm = £2.14, 15 cm × 15 cm = £4.05

SeaSorb® Soft Filler, calcium sodium alginate fibre, highly absorbent, gelling filler, 44 cm = £2.52

Sorbalgon® (Hartmann)

Calcium alginate dressing, 5 cm × 5 cm = 74p, 10 cm × 10 cm = £1.55; cavity dressing, 2 g, 32 cm = £3.17

Sorbsan® (Unomedical)

Sorbsan® Flat, calcium alginate fibre, highly absorbent, flat non-woven pads, 5 cm × 5 cm = 78p, 10 cm × 10 cm = £1.64, 10 cm × 20 cm = £3.08

Sorbsan® Plus, alginate dressing bonded to a secondary absorbent viscose pad, 7.5 cm × 10 cm = £1.66, 10 cm × 15 cm = £2.93, 10 cm × 20 cm = £3.74, 15 cm × 20 cm = £5.20

Sorbsan® Plus SA, alginate dressing with adhesive border and absorbent backing, 11.5 cm × 14 cm = £2.89, 14 cm × 19 cm = £4.22, 14 cm × 24 cm = £5.10, 19 cm × 24 cm = £6.40

Sorbsan® Ribbon, 40 cm (with probe) = £1.99

Sorbsan® Surgical Packing, 30 cm (2 g, with probe) = £3.41

Suprasorb® A (Activa)
Calcium alginate dressing, 5 cm × 5 cm = 57p, 10 cm × 10 cm = £1.12; cavity dressing, 2 g × 30 cm = £2.08

Tegaderm® Alginate (3M)
5 cm × 5 cm = 77p, 10 cm × 10 cm = £1.62; cavity dressing, 2 cm × 30 cm = £2.70

Tielle® Packing (Systagenix)
Tielle® Packing, 9.5 cm × 9.5 cm = £2.08

Urgosorb® (Urgo)
Alginate and hydrocolloid dressing without adhesive border, 5 cm × 5 cm = 81p, 10 cm × 10 cm = £1.93, 10 cm × 20 cm = £3.55; cavity dressing, 30 cm = £2.58

A8.2.7 Capillary-action dressings

Capillary-action dressings consist of an absorbent core of hydrophilic fibres sandwiched between two low-adherent wound-contact layers to ensure no fibres are shed on to the wound surface. Wound exudate is taken up by the dressing and retained within the highly absorbent central layer.

The dressing may be applied intact to relatively superficial areas, but for deeper wounds or cavities it may be cut to shape to ensure good contact with the wound base. Multiple layers may be applied to heavily exuding wounds to further increase the fluid-absorbing capacity of the dressing. A secondary adhesive dressing is necessary.

Capillary-action dressings are suitable for use on all types of exuding wounds, but particularly on sloughy wounds where removal of fluid from the wound aids debridement; capillary-action dressings are contra-indicated for heavily bleeding wounds or arterial bleeding.

Advadraw® (Advancis)
Non-adherent dressing consisting of a soft viscose and polyester absorbent pad with central wicking layer between two perforated permeable wound contact layers. 5 cm × 7.5 cm = 56p, 10 cm × 10 cm = 87p, 10 cm × 15 cm = £1.17, 15 cm × 20 cm = £1.54

Advadraw Spiral®, 0.5 cm × 40 cm = 81p

Cerdak® Basic (CliniMed)
Non-adhesive wound contact sachet containing ceramic spheres, 5 cm × 5 cm = 70p, 10 cm × 10 cm = £1.56, 10 cm × 15 cm = £2.08; cavity dressing, 10 cm × 10 cm = £2.10, 10 cm × 15 cm = £2.03

Cerdak® Aerocloth, non-adhesive wound contact sachet containing ceramic spheres, with non-woven fabric adhesive backing, 5 cm × 5 cm = £1.37, 5 cm × 10 cm = £1.94

Cerdak® Aerofilm, non-adhesive wound contact sachet containing ceramic spheres, with waterproof transparent adhesive film backing, 5 cm × 5 cm = £1.51, 5 cm × 10 cm = £2.07

Sumar® (Lantor)
Sumar® Lite, for light to moderately exuding wounds and cavities, 5 cm × 5 cm = 93p, 10 cm × 10 cm = £1.59, 10 cm × 15 cm = £2.12

Sumar® Max, for heavily exuding wounds, 5 cm × 5 cm = 95p, 10 cm × 10 cm = £1.61, 10 cm × 15 cm = £2.15

Sumar® Spiral, 0.5 cm × 40 cm = £1.57

Vacutex® (Protex)
Low-adherent dressing consisting of two external polyester wound contact layers with central wicking polyester/cotton mix absorbent layer. 5 cm × 5 cm = 94p, 10 cm × 10 cm = £1.66, 10 cm × 15 cm = £2.23, 10 cm × 20 cm = £2.68, 15 cm × 20 cm = £3.14, 20 cm × 20 cm = £4.28

A8.2.8 Odour absorbent dressings

Dressings containing activated charcoal are used to absorb odour from wounds. The underlying cause of wound odour should be identified. Wound odour is most effectively reduced by debridement of slough, reduction in bacterial levels, and frequent dressing changes.

Fungating wounds and chronic infected wounds produce high volumes of exudate. Many odour absorbent dressings are intended for use in combination with other dressings; odour absorbent dressings with a suitable wound contact layer can be used as a primary dressing.

Askina® Carbosorb (Braun)
Activated charcoal and non-woven viscose rayon dressing, 10 cm × 10 cm = £2.72, 10 cm × 20 cm = £5.25

CarboFLEX® (ConvaTec)
Dressing in 5 layers: wound-facing absorbent layer containing alginate and hydrocolloid; water-resistant second layer; third layer containing activated charcoal; non-woven absorbent fourth layer; water-resistant backing layer. 10 cm × 10 cm = £2.95, 8 cm × 15 cm = £3.55, 15 cm × 20 cm = £6.72

Carbopad® VC (Synergy Healthcare)
Activated charcoal non-absorbent dressing, 10 cm × 10 cm = £1.59, 10 cm × 20 cm = £2.15

CliniSorb® Odour Control Dressings (CliniMed)
Activated charcoal cloth enclosed in viscose rayon with outer polyamide coating. 10 cm × 10 cm = £1.75, 10 cm × 20 cm = £2.33, 15 cm × 25 cm = £3.75

Lyofoam® C (Medlock)
Lyofoam sheet with layer of activated charcoal cloth and additional outer envelope of polyurethane foam. 10 cm × 10 cm = £2.85, 15 cm × 20 cm = £6.47

Sorbsan® Plus Carbon (Unomedical)
Alginate dressing with activated carbon, 7.5 cm × 10 cm = £2.42, 10 cm × 15 cm = £4.70, 10 cm × 20 cm = £5.62, 15 cm × 20 cm = £6.47

A8.3 Antimicrobial dressings

Spreading infection at the wound site requires treatment with systemic antibacterials.

For local wound infection, a topical antimicrobial dressing can be used to reduce the level of bacteria at the wound surface but will not eliminate a spreading infection. Some dressings are designed to release the antimicrobial into the wound, others act upon the bacteria after absorption from the wound. The amount of exudate present and the level of infection should be taken into account when selecting an antimicrobial dressing.

Medical grade honey (section A8.3.1), has anti-microbial and anti-inflammatory properties. Dressings impregnated with **iodine** (section A8.3.2), can be used to treat clinically infected wounds. Dressings containing **silver** (section A8.3.3), should be used only when clinical signs or symptoms of infection are present.

Dressings containing other **antimicrobials** (section A8.3.4) such as polihexanide (polyhexamethylene biguanide) or dialkylcarbamoyl chloride are available for use on infected wounds. Although hypersensitivity is unlikely with chlorhexidine impregnated tulle dressing, the antibacterial efficacy of these dressings has not been established.

A8.3.1 Honey

Medical grade honey has antimicrobial and anti-inflammatory properties and can be used for acute or chronic wounds. Medical grade honey has osmotic properties, producing an environment that promotes autolytic debridement; it can help control wound malodour. Honey dressings should not be used on patients with extreme sensitivity to honey, bee stings or bee products. Patients with diabetes should be monitored for changes in blood-glucose concentrations during treatment with topical honey or honey-impregnated dressings.

◢**Sheet dressing**
Actilite® (Advancis)
Knitted viscose impregnated with medical grade manuka honey and manuka oil, 10 cm × 10 cm = 95p, 10 cm × 20 cm = £1.85

Activon Tulle® (Advancis)
Knitted viscose impregnated with medical grade manuka honey, 5 cm × 5 cm = £1.78, 10 cm × 10 cm = £3.01
Where no size stated by the prescriber the 5 cm size to be supplied

Algivon® (Advancis)
Absorbent, non-adherent calcium alginate dressing impregnated with medical grade manuka honey, 5 cm × 5 cm = £2.09, 10 cm × 10 cm = £3.53

Medihoney® (Medihoney)
Antibacterial Honey Tulle, woven fabric impregnated with medical grade manuka honey, 10 cm × 10 cm = £2.98
Gel sheet, sodium alginate dressing impregnated with medical grade honey, 5 cm × 5 cm = £1.75, 10 cm × 10 cm = £4.20

Mesitran® (Unomedical)
Hydrogel, semi-permeable dressing impregnated with medical grade honey, 10 cm × 10 cm = £2.51, 10 cm × 17.5 cm = £4.52, 15 cm × 20 cm = £5.22; *with adhesive border*, 10 cm × 10 cm = £2.61, 15 cm × 13 cm (sacral) = £4.42, 15 cm × 15 cm = £4.62
Mesitran® Mesh, hydrogel, non-adherent wound contact layer, without adhesive border, 10 cm × 10 cm = £2.41

◢**Honey-based topical application**
Medical grade honey is applied directly to the wound and covered with a primary low adherence wound dressing; an additional secondary dressing may be required for exuding wounds.

Activon® (Advancis)
Manuka honey, (medical grade), 25-g tube = £1.99

Medihoney® (Medihoney)
Antibacterial Medical Honey, honey (medical grade, *Leptospermum* sp.), 20-g tube = £3.96, 50-g tube = £9.90

Antibacterial Wound Gel, honey (medical grade, *Leptospermum* sp.), 80% in natural waxes and oils, 10-g tube = £2.69, 20-g tube = £4.02
Note *Antibacterial Wound Gel* is not recommended for use in deep wounds or body cavities where removal of waxes may be difficult

Melladerm® (Danetre)
Honey (medical grade; S. African, Fynbos) 45% in basis containing polyethylene glycol, 50-g tube = £7.50
Melladerm® Plus, honey (medical grade; Bulgarian, mountain flower) 45% in basis containing polyethylene glycol, 20-g tube = £4.49, 50-g tube = £8.50

Mesitran® (Unomedical)
Ointment, honey (medical grade) 47%, 15-g tube = £3.47, 50-g tube = £9.55
Excipients include lanolin

Ointment S, honey (medical grade) 40%, 15-g tube = £3.46
Excipients include lanolin

A8.3.2 Iodine

Cadexomer–iodine, like povidone–iodine, releases free iodine when exposed to wound exudate. The free iodine acts as an antiseptic on the wound surface, the cadexomer absorbs wound exudate and encourages desloughing.

Two-component hydrogel dressings containing glucose oxidase and iodide ions generate a low level of free iodine in the presence of moisture and oxygen.

Povidone–iodine fabric dressing is a knitted viscose dressing with povidone–iodine incorporated in a hydrophilic polyethylene glycol basis; this facilitates diffusion of the iodine into the wound and permits removal of the dressing by irrigation. The iodine has a wide spectrum of antimicrobial activity but it is rapidly deactivated by wound exudate.

Systemic absorption of iodine may occur, particularly from large wounds or with prolonged use.

Iodoflex® (S&N Hlth.)
Paste, iodine 0.9% as cadexomer–iodine in a paste basis with gauze backing, 5-g unit = £3.73; 10 g = £7.46; 17 g = £11.81
Uses for treatment of chronic exuding wounds; max. single application 50 g; max. weekly application 150 g; max. duration up to 3 months in any single course of treatment
Cautions iodine may be absorbed, particularly from large wounds or during prolonged use; severe renal impairment; history of thyroid disorder
Contra-indications children; patients receiving lithium; thyroid disorders; pregnancy and breast-feeding

Iodosorb® (S&N Hlth.)
Ointment, iodine 0.9% as cadexomer–iodine in an ointment basis, 10 g = £4.04; 20 g = £8.24
Powder, iodine 0.9% as cadexomer–iodine microbeads, 3-g sachet = £1.76
Uses for treatment of chronic exuding wounds; max. single application 50 g; max. weekly application 150 g; max. duration up to 3 months in any single course of treatment
Cautions iodine may be absorbed, particularly from large wounds or during prolonged use; severe renal impairment; history of thyroid disorder
Contra-indications children; patients receiving lithium; thyroid disorders; pregnancy and breast-feeding

Iodozyme® (Insense)
Hydrogel (two-component dressing containing glucose oxidase and iodide ions), 10 cm × 10 cm = £12.50
Uses antimicrobial dressing for lightly to moderately exuding wounds
Cautions children; pregnancy and breast-feeding
Contra-indications thyroid disorders; patients receiving lithium

Oxyzyme® (Insense)

Hydrogel (two-component dressing containing glucose oxidase and iodide ions), 6.5 cm × 5 cm = £6.00, 10 cm × 10 cm = £10.00

Uses non-infected, dry to moderately exuding wounds

Cautions children; pregnancy and breast-feeding

Contra-indications thyroid disorders; patients receiving lithium

Povidone–iodine Fabric Dressing

(Drug Tariff specification 43). Knitted viscose primary dressing impregnated with povidone–iodine ointment 10%, 5 cm × 5 cm = 32p; 9.5 cm × 9.5 cm = 47p (Systagenix—*Inadine®*)

Uses wound contact layer for abrasions and superficial burns

Cautions iodine may be absorbed particularly if large wounds treated; children under 6 months; thyroid disease

Contra-indications severe renal impairment; pregnancy; breast-feeding

A8.3.3 Silver

Antimicrobial dressings containing **silver** should be used only when infection is suspected as a result of clinical signs or symptoms (see also p. 41). Silver ions exert an antimicrobial effect in the presence of wound exudate; the volume of wound exudate as well as the presence of infection should be considered when selecting a silver-containing dressing.

Dressings impregnated with silver sulfadiazine have broad antimicrobial activity; if silver sulfadiazine is applied to large areas, or used for prolonged periods, there is a risk of blood disorders and skin discolouration (see BNF section 13.10.1.1). The use of silver sulfadiazine-impregnated dressings is contra-indicated in neonates, in pregnancy, and in patients with significant renal or hepatic impairment.

◢**Low adherence dressings**

Acticoat® (S&N Hlth.)

Three layer antimicrobial barrier dressing consisting of a polyester core between low adherent silver coated high density polyethylene mesh, 5 cm × 5 cm = £3.22, 10 cm × 10 cm = £7.85, 10 cm × 20 cm = £12.28, 20 cm × 40 cm = £42.01

Acticoat® 7 five layer antimicrobial barrier dressing consisting of a polyester core between low adherent silver coated high density polyethylene mesh, 5 cm × 5 cm = £5.59, 10 cm × 12.5 cm = £16.65, 15 cm × 15 cm = £29.93

Atrauman® Ag (Hartmann)

Non-adherent polyamide fabric impregnated with silver and neutral triglycerides, 5 cm × 5 cm = 47p, 10 cm × 10 cm = £1.14, 10 cm × 20 cm = £2.23

◢**With charcoal**

Actisorb® Silver 220 (Systagenix)

Knitted fabric of activated charcoal, with one-way stretch, with silver residues, within spun-bonded nylon sleeve. 6.5 cm × 9.5 cm = £1.61, 10.5 cm × 10.5 cm = £2.53, 10.5 cm × 19 cm = £4.60

◢**Soft polymer dressings**

Mepilex® Ag (Mölnlycke)

Soft silicone wound contact dressing with polyurethane foam film backing, with silver, 10 cm × 10 cm = £5.80, 10 cm × 20 cm = £9.57, 15 cm × 15 cm = £10.77, 20 cm × 20 cm = £15.96

UrgoCell® Silver (Urgo)

Non-adherent soft polymer wound contact dressing with polyurethane foam film backing, with silver, 6 cm × 6 cm = £4.00, 10 cm × 10 cm = £5.50, 15 cm × 20 cm = £9.90

Urgotul® Silver (Urgo)

Non-adherent soft polymer wound contact dressing, with silver, 10 cm × 12 cm = £3.32, 15 cm × 20 cm = £9.03

Urgotul® Duo Silver, non-adherent, soft polymer wound contact dressing, with silver, 5 cm × 7 cm = £1.94, 11 cm × 11 cm = £3.85, 15 cm × 20 cm = £9.28

◢**Hydrocolloid dressings**

Aquacel® Ag (ConvaTec)

Soft non-woven pad containing hydrocolloid fibres, (silver impregnated), 4 cm × 10 cm = £2.65, 4 cm × 20 cm = £3.46, 4 cm × 30 cm = £5.17, 5 cm × 5 cm = £1.81, 10 cm × 10 cm = £4.32, 15 cm × 15 cm = £8.13, 20 cm × 30 cm = £20.17; 2 cm × 45 cm (ribbon) = £4.34

Biatain® Ag Hydrocolloid (Coloplast)

Semi-permeable, antimicrobial barrier dressing with ionic silver (silver sodium thiosulphate), 10 cm × 10 cm = £6.72, 15 cm × 15 cm = £13.44

Physiotulle® Ag (Coloplast)

Non-adherent polyester fabric with hydrocolloid and silver sulfadiazine, 10 cm × 10 cm = £2.10

Urgotul® SSD (Urgo)

Non-adherent, polyester fabric with hydrocolloid and silver sulfadiazine, 11 cm × 11 cm = £2.97, 16 cm × 21 cm = £8.42

Contra-indications pregnancy, renal, or hepatic impairment, neonates

◢**Foam dressings**

Acticoat® Moisture Control (S&N Hlth.)

Three layer polyurethane dressing consisting of a silver coated layer, a foam layer, and a waterproof layer, 5 cm × 5 cm = £6.58, 10 cm × 10 cm = £15.39, 10 cm × 20 cm = £29.99

Allevyn® Ag (S&N Hlth.)

Silver sulfadiazine impregnated polyurethane foam film dressing *with adhesive border*, 7.5 cm × 7.5 cm = £3.21, 10 cm × 10 cm = £5.06, 12.5 cm × 12.5 cm = £6.65, 17.5 cm × 17.5 cm = £12.79, 17 cm × 17 cm (sacral) = £9.99, 22 cm × 22 cm (sacral) = £13.38; *without adhesive border*, 5 cm × 5 cm = £3.00, 10 cm × 10 cm = £5.65, 15 cm × 15 cm = £10.71, 20 cm × 20 cm = £15.69, 10.5 cm × 13.5 cm (heel) = £9.90

Cautions large open wounds; sensitivity to sulphonamides; G6PD deficiency; significant hepatic or renal impairment; **interactions**: Appendix 1 (sulphonamides)

Avance® (Medlock)

Silver impregnated polyurethane foam film dressing, *without adhesive border*, 10 cm × 10 cm = £2.75, 10 cm × 17.5 cm = £4.38, 15 cm × 20 cm = £6.05; *with adhesive border*, 9 cm × 9 cm = £2.31, 12 cm × 12 cm = £3.83, 15 cm × 15 cm = £4.69, 15 cm × 13 cm (sacral) = £3.45

Biatain® Ag (Coloplast)

Silver impregnated polyurethane foam film dressing *with adhesive border*, 12.5 cm × 12.5 cm = £8.55, 18 cm × 18 cm = £17.14, 19 cm × 20 cm (heel) = £16.91, 23 cm × 23 cm (sacral) = £17.97; *without adhesive border*, 10 cm × 10 cm = £7.47, 5 cm × 7 cm = £3.07, 10 cm × 20 cm = £13.73, 15 cm × 15 cm = £15.00, 20 cm × 20 cm = £21.15, 5 cm diameter = £3.13; cavity dressing 5 cm × 8 cm = £3.72

PolyMem® (Unomedical)

Silver impregnated polyurethane foam film dressing, *with adhesive border*, 5 cm × 7.6 cm (oval) = £2.15, 12.7 cm × 8.8 cm (oval) = £5.30; *without adhesive border*, 10.8 cm × 10.8 cm = £8.20, 17 cm × 19 cm = £16.93

◢**Alginate dressings**

Acticoat® Absorbent (S&N Hlth.)

Calcium alginate dressing with a silver coated antimicrobial barrier, 5 cm × 5 cm = £4.91, 10 cm × 12.5 cm = £11.78; 2 cm × 30 cm (cavity) = £11.85

Algisite® Ag (S&N Hlth.)

Calcium alginate dressing, with silver, 5 cm × 5 cm = £1.53, 10 cm × 10 cm = £3.83, 10 cm × 20 cm = £7.04; 2 g, 30 cm (cavity) = £5.28

Silvercel® (Systagenix)

Alginate and hydrocolloid dressing impregnated with silver, 2.5 cm × 30.5 cm = £4.37, 5 cm × 5 cm = £1.64, 10 cm × 20 cm = £7.53, 11 cm × 11 cm = £4.06

Sorbsan® (Unomedical)

Sorbsan® Silver Flat, calcium alginate fibre, highly absorbent, flat non-woven pads, with silver, 5 cm × 5 cm = £1.50, 10 cm × 10 cm = £3.80, 10 cm × 20 cm = £6.94

Sorbsan® Silver Plus, calcium alginate dressing with absorbent backing, with silver, 7.5 cm × 10 cm = £3.25, 10 cm × 15 cm = £5.41, 10 cm × 20 cm = £6.58, 15 cm × 20 cm = £8.82

Sorbsan® Silver Plus SA, calcium alginate dressing with absorbent backing and adhesive border, with silver, 11.5 cm × 14 cm = £5.28, 14 cm × 19 cm = £7.60, 14 cm × 24 cm = £8.36, 19 cm × 24 cm = £9.32

Sorbsan® Silver Ribbon, with silver, 40 cm (with probe) = £3.97

Sorbsan® Silver Surgical Packing, with silver, 30 cm (2 g, with probe) = £5.55

Urgosorb® Silver (Urgo)

Alginate and hydrocolloid dressing, impregnated with silver, 5 cm × 5 cm = £1.42, 10 cm × 10 cm = £3.39, 10 cm × 20 cm = £6.39; cavity dressing, 2.5 cm × 30 cm = £3.41

A8.3.4 Other antimicrobials

Chlorhexidine Gauze Dressing, BP 1993

Fabric of leno weave, weft and warp threads of cotton and/or viscose yarn, impregnated with ointment containing chlorhexidine acetate, 5 cm × 5 cm = 27p; 10 cm × 10 cm = 56p (S&N Hlth.—Bactigras®)

Cutimed® Sorbact (BSN Medical)

Low adherence acetate tissue impregnated with dialkylcarbamoyl chloride, (dressing pad) 7 cm × 9 cm = £3.20, 10 cm × 10 cm = £5.00, 10 cm × 20 cm = £7.80; (swabs) 4 cm × 6 cm = £1.50, 7 cm × 9 cm = £2.50, (round swabs) 3 cm, 5 pad pack = £3.00; (cavity dressing, cotton) 2 cm × 50 cm = £3.74, 5 cm × 2 m = £7.37

Flaminal® (Ark Therapeutics)

Forte gel, alginate with glucose oxidase and lactoperoxidase, for moderately to heavily exuding wounds, 15 g = £7.18, 50 g = £23.77

Hydro gel, alginate with glucose oxidase and lactoperoxidase, for lightly to moderately exuding wounds, 15 g = £7.18, 50 g = £23.77

Prontosan® Wound Gel (Braun)

Hydrogel containing betaine surfactant and polyhexanide, 30 mL = £5.97

Suprasorb® X + PHMB (Activa)

Biosynthetic cellulose fibre dressing with polihexanide, 5 cm × 5 cm = £2.34, 9 cm × 9 cm = £4.66, 14 cm × 20 cm = £10.60; 2 cm × 21 cm (rope) = £6.60

Telfa® AMD (Covidien)

Low adherence absorbent perforated plastic film faced dressing with polihexanide, 7.5 cm × 10 cm = 17p, 7.5 cm × 20 cm = 28p

Telfa® AMD Island Low adherence dressing with adhesive border and absorbent pad, with polihexanide, 10 cm × 12.5 cm = 58p, 10 cm × 20 cm = 85p, 10 cm × 25.5 cm = 96p, 10 cm × 35 cm = £1.19

A8.4 Specialised dressings

A8.4.1 Protease-modulating matrix dressings

Protease-modulating matrix dressings alter the activity of *proteolytic enzymes* in chronic wounds; the clinical significance of this approach is yet to be demonstrated.

Cadesorb® (S&N Hlth.)

Ointment, starch-based, 10 g = £4.96, 20 g = £8.46

Promogran® (Systagenix)

Collagen and oxidised regenerated cellulose matrix, applied directly to wound and covered with suitable dressing, 28 cm^2 (hexagonal) = £5.09, 123 cm^2 (hexagonal) = £15.32

Promogran® Prisma® Matrix (Systagenix)

Collagen, silver and oxidised regenerated cellulose matrix, applied directly to wound and covered with suitable dressing, 28 cm^2 (hexagonal) = £6.19, 123 cm^2 (hexagonal) = £17.63

Sorbion® S (H&R)

Absorbent polymers in cellulose matrix, hypoallergenic fleece envelope, 7.5 cm × 7.5 cm = £1.75, 10 cm × 10 cm = £2.22, 20 cm × 20 cm = £6.90, 20 cm × 10 cm = £3.68, 30 cm × 10 cm = £5.29, 30 cm × 20 cm = £9.92, 12 cm × 5 cm = £1.86

Suprasorb® C (Activa)

Collagen, 4 cm × 6 cm = £2.60, 6 cm × 8 cm = £3.98, 8 cm × 12 cm = £7.80

Tegaderm® Matrix (3M)

Cellulose acetate matrix, impregnated with polyhydrated ionogens ointment in polyethylene glycol basis, 5 cm × 6 cm = £4.75, 8 cm × 10 cm = £9.75

A8.4.2 Silicone keloid dressings

Silicone gel and gel sheets are used to reduce or prevent hypertrophic and keloid scarring. They should not be used on open wounds. Application times should be increased gradually. Silicone sheets can be washed and reused.

Advasil® Conform (Advancis)

Self-adhesive silicone gel sheet with polyurethane film backing, 10 cm × 10 cm = £5.20, 10 cm × 15 cm = £9.17

Cica-Care® (S&N Hlth.)

Soft, self-adhesive, semi-occlusive silicone gel sheet with backing. 6 cm × 12 cm = £13.42; 15 cm × 12 cm = £26.16

Ciltech® (Su-Med)

Silicone gel sheet, 10 cm × 10 cm = £7.50, 15 cm × 15 cm = £14.00, 10 cm × 20 cm = £12.50

Silicone gel, 15 g = £17.50, 60 g = £50.00

Dermatix® (Valeant)

Self-adhesive silicone gel sheet (clear- or fabric-backed), 4 cm × 13 cm = £6.61, 13 cm × 15 cm = £15.17, 13 cm × 25 cm = £27.41, 20 cm × 30 cm = £49.92; Silicone gel, 15 g = £19.38, 60 g = £58.14

Kelo-cote® (ABT Healthcare)

Silicone gel, 15 g = £17.88, 60 g = £51.00

Silicone spray, 100 mL = £51.00

Mepiform® (Mölnlycke)

Self-adhesive silicone gel sheet with polyurethane film backing, 5 cm × 7 cm = £3.20, 9 cm × 18 cm = £12.53, 4 cm × 31 cm = £10.12

Silgel® (Nagor)

Silicone gel sheet, 10 cm × 10 cm = £13.50; 20 cm × 20 cm = £40.00; 40 cm × 40 cm = £144.00; 10 cm × 5 cm = £7.50; 15 cm x 10 cm = £19.50; 30 cm × 5 cm = £19.50; 10 cm × 30 cm = £31.50; 25 cm × 15 cm (submammary) = £21.12; 46 cm × 8.5 cm (abdominal) = £39.46; 5.5 cm diameter (circular) = £4.00

Silgel® STC-SE silicone gel, 20-mL tube = £19.00

A8.5   Adjunct dressings and appliances

A8.5.1   Surgical absorbents

Surgical absorbent dressings, applied directly to the wound, have many disadvantages, since they adhere to the wound, shed fibres into it, and dehydrate it; they also permit leakage of exudate ('strike through') with an associated risk of infection. Surgical absorbents may be used as secondary absorbent layers in the management of heavily exuding wounds.

◢ Cotton

Absorbent Cotton, BP

Carded cotton fibres of not less than 10 mm average staple length, available in rolls and balls, 25 g = 69p; 100 g = £1.58; 500 g = £5.31 (most suppliers). 25-g pack to be supplied when weight not stated

Uses general purpose cleansing and swabbing, pre-operative skin preparation, application of medicaments; supplementary absorbent pad to absorb excess wound exudate

Absorbent Cotton, Hospital Quality

As for absorbent cotton but lower quality materials, shorter staple length etc. 100 g = £1.10; 500 g = £3.46 (most suppliers)

Drug Tariff specifies to be supplied only where specifically ordered

Uses suitable only as general purpose absorbent, for swabbing, and routine cleansing of incontinent patients; not for wound cleansing

◢ Gauze and tissue

Absorbent Cotton Gauze, BP 1988

Cotton fabric of plain weave, in rolls and as swabs (see below), usually Type 13 light, sterile, 90 cm (all) × 1 m = £1.04; 3 m = £2.17; 5 m = £3.38; 10 m = £6.47 (most suppliers). 1-m packet supplied when no size stated

Uses pre-operative preparation, for cleansing and swabbing

Note Drug Tariff also includes unsterilised absorbent cotton gauze, 25 m roll = £14.82

Absorbent Cotton Ribbon Gauze, BP 1993 ⟨JHS⟩

Cotton fabric of plain weave in ribbon form with fast selvedge edges

Uses post-surgery cavity packing for sinus, dental, throat cavities etc.

Absorbent Cotton and Viscose Ribbon Gauze, BP 1993

Woven fabric in ribbon form with fast selvedge edges, warp threads of cotton, weft threads of viscose or combined cotton and viscose yarn, sterile. 5 m (both) × 1.25 cm = 78p; 2.5 cm = 86p

Uses post-surgery cavity packing for sinus, dental, throat cavities etc.

Gauze and Cotton Tissue, BP 1988

Consists of absorbent cotton enclosed in absorbent cotton gauze type 12 or absorbent cotton and viscose gauze type 2. 500 g = £6.74 (most suppliers, including Robinsons—Gamgee Tissue® (blue label))

Uses absorbent and protective pad, as burns dressing on non-adherent layer

Gauze and Cotton Tissue

(Drug Tariff specification 14). Similar to above. 500 g = £4.92 (most suppliers, including Robinsons—Gamgee Tissue® (pink label))

Drug Tariff specifies to be supplied only where specifically ordered

Uses absorbent and protective pad, as burns dressing on non-adherent layer

◢ Lint and muslin

Absorbent Lint, BPC ◢

Cotton cloth of plain weave with nap raised on one side from warp threads. 25 g = 86p; 100 g = £2.63; 500 g = £11.07 (most suppliers). 25-g pack supplied where no quantity stated

Note Not recommended for wound management

Absorbent Muslin, BP 1988 ⟨JHS⟩

Fabric of plain weave, warp threads of cotton, weft threads of cotton and/or viscose

Uses wet dressing, soaked in 0.9% sterile sodium chloride solution

◢ Pads

Absorbent Dressing Pads, Sterile

Drisorb®, 10 cm × 20 cm = 17p (Synergy Healthcare)

Xupad®, 10 cm × 20 cm = 17p, 20 cm × 20 cm = 28p, 20 cm × 40 cm = 40p (Richardson)

[1] Surgipad® (Systagenix) ⟨JHS⟩

Absorbent pad of absorbent cotton and viscose in sleeve of non-woven viscose fabric, pouch 12 cm × 10 cm = 18p, 20 cm × 10 cm = 25p, 20 cm × 20 cm = 30p, 40 cm × 20 cm = 41p; non sterile pack 12 cm × 10 cm = 5p, 20 cm × 10 cm = 10p, 20 cm × 20 cm = 17p, 40 cm × 20 cm = 28p

1. ⟨JHS⟩ Except in Sterile Dressing Pack with Non-woven Pads

A8.5.2   Wound drainage pouches

Biotrol® (Braun)

Draina S Fistula, wound drainage pouch, mini (cut to 20 mm), 150-mL capacity = £2.40; medium (cut to 50 mm), 350-mL capacity = £3.59; large (cut to 88 mm), 500-mL capacity = £4.41

Draina S Vision, wound drainage pouch, (cut to 50 mm), 150-mL capacity = £9.39; (cut to 88 mm), 250-mL capacity = £9.92; (cut to 100 mm), 300-mL capacity = £11.51

Dermasure® (ADI Medical)

Pouch, small (wound size up to 9 cm × 16 cm) = £15.60; medium (wound size up to 15 cm × 27 cm) ■ £20.00

Eakin® (Eakin)

Wound pouch, fold and tuck closure, small (wound size up to 45 mm × 30 mm) = £4.50; medium (wound size up to 110 mm × 75 mm) = £6.50; large (wound size up to 175 mm × 110 mm) = £8.50; extra large (horizontal wound up to 245 mm × 160 mm) = £15.00

Wound pouch, bung closure, small (wound size up to 45 mm × 30 mm) = £5.00; medium (wound size up to 110 mm × 75 mm) = £7.00; large (wound size up to 175 mm × 110 mm) = £9.50; extra large (horizontal or vertical wound up to 245 mm × 160 mm) = £17.00, (vertical incision wound up to 290 mm × 130 mm) = £17.00; (horizontal wound up to 245 mm × 160 mm), with access window = £19.00

Access window, for use with Eakin® pouches = £7.00

Oakmed® Option (Oakmed)

Wound Manager, extra small (wound size up to 90 mm × 180 mm) = £10.91; small (horizontal wound size up to 245 mm × 160 mm) = £12.13; medium (vertical wound size up to 90 mm × 260 mm) = £12.41; large (wound size up to 160 mm × 200 mm) = £12.95

Wound manager, with access port, extra small (wound size up to 90 mm × 180 mm) = £11.93; small (horizontal wound size up to 245 mm × 160 mm) = £12.68; medium (vertical wound size up to 90 mm × 260 mm) = £12.95; large (wound size up to 160 mm × 260 mm) = £15.81; square (vertical wound size up to 160 mm × 200 mm) = £13.49

Wound manager, cut-to-fit, small (10–30 mm) = £2.23, medium (10–50 mm) = £2.47, large (10–50 mm) = £2.59

Welland® (CliniMed)

Fistula bag, *wound manager*, cut-to-fit (wound size up ro 40 mm × 70 mm) = £2.54

A8.6 Complex adjunct therapies

Topical negative pressure (or vacuum-assisted) therapy requires specific wound dressings for use with the vacuum-pump equipment.

Other complex adjunct therapies include sterile larvae (maggots), and growth factors such as becalpermin (see BNF section 13.11.7)

A8.6.1 Topical negative pressure therapy

◀**Vacuum assisted closure products**
Exsu-Fast® (Synergy Healthcare)

Dressing kit, Kit 1 (small wound, low exudate) = £28.04; Kit 2 (large wound, heavy exudate) = £35.83; Kit 3 (large wound, medium to low exudate) = £35.83; Kit 4 (small wound, heavy exudate) = £28.04

V.A.C. GranuFoam® (KCI Medical)

Dressing kit, polyurethane foam dressing (with adhesive drapes and pad connector), 10 cm × 7.5 cm × 3.3 cm (small) = £21.41, 18 cm × 12.5 cm × 3.3 cm (medium) = £25.49, 26 cm × 15 cm × 3.3 cm (large) = £29.57

Venturi® (Talley)

Wound sealing kit, flat drain, standard = £15.00, large = £17.50; channel drain = £15.00

V1STA® (S&N Hlth.)

Dressing kit, flat drain, small = £16.52, medium = £20.70, large = £26.28; round drain, small = £16.52, large = £26.28; channel drain, medium = £20.70

WoundASSIST® (Huntleigh)

Wound pack, small–medium = £20.50, medium–large = £23.50

◀**Wound drainage collection devices**
V.A.C Freedom® (KCI Medical)

Canister (with gel), 300 mL = £26.51

Venturi® (Talley)

Canister kit (with solidifier) = £12.50

V1STA® (S&N Hlth.)

Canister kit, 250 mL (with solidifier) = £18.63, 800 mL (with solidifier) = £20.70

WoundASSIST® (Huntleigh)

Canister, 500 mL = £20.00

A8.7 Wound care acccessories

A8.7.1 Dressing packs

The role of dressing packs is very limited. They are used to provide a clean or sterile working surface; some packs shown below include cotton wool balls, which are not recommended for use on wounds.

Non-Drug Tariff Specification Sterile Dressing Pack

Dressit® contains vitrex gloves, large apron, disposable bag, paper towel, softswabs, adsorbent pad, sterile field = 60p (Richardson)

Nurse It® contains powder-free vinyl gloves, sterile polythene sheet, non-woven swabs, paper towel, disposable bag, compartmented tray, plastic forceps = 52p (Medicare)

Polyfield® Nitrile Patient Pack contains powder-free nitrile gloves, laminate sheet, non-woven swabs, towel, polythene disposable bag, apron = 52p (Shermond)

Polyfield® Soft Vinyl Patient Pack contains powder-free sterile soft vinyl gloves, polythene sheet, non-woven swabs, towel, polythene disposable bag, apron = 52p (Shermond)

Propax® SDP contains paper towel, disposable bag, gauze swabs, dressing pad, sterile field = 45p (BSN Medical)

Woundcare® contains nitrile gloves, sterile field, compartmented tray, large apron, disposable bag, non-woven swabs, drape = 44p (Frontier)

Sterile Dressing Pack

(Drug Tariff specification 10). Contains gauze and cotton tissue pad, gauze swabs, absorbent cotton wool balls, absorbent paper towel, water repellent inner wrapper. 1 pack = 49p (Synergy Healthcare—*Vernaid®*)

Sterile Dressing Pack with Non-woven Pads

(Drug Tariff specification 35). Contains non-woven fabric covered dressing pad, non-woven fabric swabs, absorbent cotton wool balls, absorbent paper towel, water repellent inner wrapper. 1 pack = 48p (Synergy Healthcare—*Vernaid®*)

A8.7.2 Woven and fabric swabs

Gauze Swab, BP 1988

Consists of absorbent cotton gauze type 13 light or absorbent cotton and viscose gauze type 1 folded into squares or rectangles of 8-ply with no cut edges exposed, sterile, 7.5 cm × 7.5 cm 5-pad packet = 38p; non-sterile, 10 cm × 10 cm, 100-pad packet = £1.31 (most suppliers)

Filmated Gauze Swab, BP 1988

As for Gauze Swab, but with thin layer of Absorbent Cotton enclosed within, non-sterile, 10 cm × 10 cm, 100-pad packet = £3.52 (Synergy Healthcare—*Cotfil®*)

Non-woven Fabric Swab

(Drug Tariff specification 28). Consists of non-woven fabric folded 4-ply; alternative to gauze swabs, type 13 light, sterile, 7.5 cm × 7.5 cm, 5-pad packet = 24p; non-sterile, 10 cm × 10 cm, 100-pad packet = 76p

Filmated Non-woven Fabric Swab

(Drug Tariff specification 29). Film of viscose fibres enclosed within non-woven viscose fabric folded 8-ply, non-sterile, 10 cm × 10 cm, 100-pad packet = £3.52 (Systagenix—*Regal®*)

A8.7.3   Surgical adhesive tapes

Adhesive tapes are useful for retaining dressings on joints or awkward body parts. These tapes, particularly those containing rubber, can cause irritant and allergic reactions in susceptible patients; synthetic adhesives have been developed to overcome this problem, but they, too, may sometimes be associated with reactions. Synthetic adhesive, or silicon adhesive, tapes can be used for patients with skin reactions to plasters and strapping containing rubber, or undergoing prolonged treatment.

Adhesive tapes that are occlusive may cause skin maceration. Care is needed not to apply these tapes under tension, to avoid creating a tourniquet effect. If applied over joints they need to be orientated so that the area of maximum extensibility of the fabric is in the direction of movement of the limb.

◢Permeable adhesive tapes
Elastic Adhesive Tape, BP 1988
(Elastic Adhesive Plaster). Woven fabric, elastic in warp (crepe-twisted cotton threads), weft of cotton and/or viscose threads, spread with adhesive mass containing zinc oxide. 4.5 m stretched × 2.5 cm = £1.64 (Robinsons—*Flexoplast*®; S&N—*Elastoplast*®)

For 5 cm width, see Elastic Adhesive Bandage

Permeable, Apertured Non-Woven Synthetic Adhesive Tape, BP 1988
Non-woven fabric with a polyacrylate adhesive.

Hypafix®, 5 cm × 5 m = £1.34, 10 cm × 5 m = £2.25, 10 m (all): 2.5 cm = £1.56, 5 cm = £2.48, 10 cm = £4.33, 15 cm = £6.42, 20 cm = £8.51, 30 cm = £12.31 (BSN Medical)

Mefix®, 5 m (all): 2.5 cm = 95p, 5 cm = £1.68; 10 cm = £2.69, 15 cm = £3.66, 20 cm = £4.69, 30 cm = £6.72 (Mölnlycke)

Omnifix®, 10 m (all): 5 cm = £2.19, 10 cm = £3.69, 15 cm = £5.44 (Hartmann)

Permeable Non-woven Synthetic Adhesive Tape, BP 1988
Backing of paper-based or non-woven textile material spread with a polymeric adhesive mass:

Clinipore®, 5 m (all) 1.25 cm = 35p, 2.5 cm = 59p, 5 cm = 99p; 2.5 cm × 10 m = 73p (Clinisupplies)

Leukofix®, 5 m (all) 1.25 cm = 52p, 2.5 cm = 83p, 5 cm = £1.45 (BSN Medical)

Leukopor®, 5 m (all) 1.25 cm = 46p, 2.5 cm = 72p, 5 cm = £1.26 (BSN Medical)

Mediplast®, 5 m (all) 1.25 cm = 30p, 2.5 cm = 50p (Neomedic)

Micropore®, 5 m (all) 1.25 cm = 60p, 2.5 cm = 89p, 5 cm = £1.57 (3M)

Scanpor®, 5 m (all) 1.25 cm = 40p, 2.5 cm = 65p, 5 cm = £1.12; 10 m (all), 1.25 cm = 52p, 2.5 cm = 87p, 5 cm = £1.65, 7.5 cm = £2.42 (BioDiagnostics)

Where no brand stated by prescriber, net price of tape supplied not to exceed 35p (1.25 cm), 59p (2.5 cm), 99p (5 cm)

Permeable Woven Synthetic Adhesive Tape, BP 1988
Non-extensible closely woven fabric, spread with a polymeric adhesive. 5 m (all): 1.25 cm = 77p; 2.5 cm = £1.12; 5 cm = £1.95 (Beiersdorf—*Leukosilk*®)

Silicone adhesive tape
Soft silicone, water-resistant, knitted fabric, polyurethane film adhesive tape

Insil®, 2 cm × 3 m = £5.60, 4 cm × 1.5 m = £5.60 (Insight)

Mepitac®, 2 cm × 3 m = £6.39, 4 cm × 1.5 m = £6.39 (Mölnlycke)

Siltape®, 2 cm × 3 m = £5.60, 4 cm × 1.5 m = £5.60 (Advancis)

Zinc Oxide Adhesive Tape, BP 1988
(Zinc Oxide Plaster). Fabric, plain weave, warp and weft of cotton and/or viscose, spread with an adhesive containing zinc oxide. 5 m (all): 1.25 cm = 93p; 2.5 cm = £1.35; 5 cm = £2.28; 7.5 cm = £3.43 (most suppliers)

Zinc Oxide Adhesive Tape
Mediplast®, 5 m (all), 1.25 cm = 82p, 2.5 cm = £1.19, 5 cm = £1.99, 7.5 cm = £2.99 (Neomedic)

Strappal®, 5 m (all): 1.25 cm = 89p, 2.5 cm = £1.29, 5 cm = £2.17, 7.5 cm = £3.27 (BSN Medical)

◢Occlusive adhesive tapes
Impermeable Plastic Adhesive Tape, BP 1988
Extensible water-impermeable plastic film spread with an adhesive mass. 2.5 cm × 3 m = £1.30; 2.5 cm × 5 m = £1.95; 5 cm × 5 m = £2.47; 7.5 cm × 5 m = £3.59 (BSN Medical—*Sleek*®)

Impermeable Plastic Synthetic Adhesive Tape, BP 1988
Extensible water-impermeable plastic film spread with a polymeric adhesive mass. 5 m (both): 2.5 cm = £1.72; 5 cm = £3.27 (3M—*Blenderm*®)

A8.7.4   Adhesive dressings

Adhesive dressings (also termed 'island dressings') have a limited role for minor wounds only. The inclusion of an antiseptic is not particularly useful and may cause skin irritation in susceptible subjects.

◢Permeable adhesive dressings
Elastic Adhesive Dressing, BP 1993 ⟨JHS⟩
Wound dressing or dressing strip, pad attached to piece of extension plaster, leaving suitable adhesive margin; both pad and margin covered with suitable protector; pad may be dyed yellow and may be impregnated with suitable antiseptic (see below); extension plaster may be perforated or ventilated

Note Permitted antiseptics are aminoacridine hydrochloride (aminacrine hydrochloride), chlorhexidine hydrochloride (both 0.07–0.13%), chlorhexidine gluconate (0.11–0.20%); domiphen bromide (0.05–0.25%)

Permeable Plastic Wound Dressing, BP 1993 ⟨JHS⟩
Consisting of an absorbent pad, which may be dyed and impregnated with a suitable antiseptic (see under Elastic Adhesive Dressing), attached to a piece of permeable plastic surgical adhesive tape, to leave a suitable adhesive margin; both pad and margin covered with suitable protector (most suppliers)

◢Vapour permeable adhesive dressings
Vapour-permeable Waterproof Plastic Wound Dressing, BP 1993
(former Drug Tariff title: Semipermeable Waterproof Plastic Wound Dressing). Consists of absorbent pad, may be dyed and impregnated with suitable antiseptic (see under Elastic Adhesive Dressing), attached to piece of semi-permeable waterproof surgical adhesive tape, to leave suitable adhesive margin; both pad and margin covered with suitable protector.(S&N Hlth—*Elastoplast Airstrip*®)

◢Occlusive adhesive tapes
Impermeable Plastic Wound Dressing, BP 1993 ⟨JHS⟩
Consists of absorbent pad, may be dyed and impregnated with suitable antiseptic (see under Elastic Adhesive Dressing), attached to piece of impermeable plastic surgical adhesive tape, to leave suitable adhesive margin; both pad and margin covered with suitable protector (most suppliers)

A8.7.5 Skin closure dressings

Skin closure strips are used as an alternative to sutures for minor cuts and lacerations. Skin tissue adhesive (BNF section 13.10.5) can be used for closure of minor skin wounds and for additional suture support.

Skin closure strips, sterile
Leukostrip®, 6.4 mm × 76 mm, 3 strips per envelope. 10 envelopes = £5.79 (S&N Hlth.)
Steri-strip®, 6 mm × 75 mm, 3 strips per envelope. 12 envelopes = £8.52 (3M)
Drug Tariff specifies that these are specifically for personal administration by the prescriber

A8.8 Bandages

According to their structure and performance bandages are used for dressing retention, for support, and for compression.

A8.8.1 Non-extensible bandages

Bandages made from non-extensible woven fabrics have generally been replaced by more conformable products, therefore their role is now extremely limited. Triangular calico bandage has a role as a sling.

Domette Bandage, BP 1988 NHS
Fabric, plain weave, cotton warp and wool weft (hospital quality also available, all cotton). 5 m (all): 5 cm = 54p; 7.5 cm = 81p; 10 cm = £1.08; 15 cm = £1.61 (Steraid)

Multiple Pack Dressing No. 1
(Drug Tariff). Contains absorbent cotton, absorbent cotton gauze type 13 light (sterile), open-wove bandages (banded). 1 pack = £3.93

Open-wove Bandage, BP 1988
Cotton cloth, plain weave, warp of cotton, weft of cotton, viscose, or combination, one continuous length. Type 1, 5 m (all): 2.5 cm = 30p; 5 cm = 51p; 7.5 cm = 72p; 10 cm = 94p (most suppliers) 5 m × 5 cm supplied when size not stated

Triangular Calico Bandage, BP 1980
Unbleached calico right-angled triangle, 90 cm × 90 cm × 1.27 m = £1.13 (most suppliers)

A8.8.2 Light-weight conforming bandages

Lightweight conforming bandages are used for dressing retention, with the aim of keeping the dressing close to the wound without inhibiting movement or restricting blood flow. The elasticity of **conforming-stretch bandages** (also termed contour bandages) is greater than that of **cotton conforming bandages**.

Conforming Bandage (Synthetic)
Fabric, plain weave, warp of polyamide, weft of viscose. 4 m stretched (all):
Hospiform® (formerly *Peha Crepp*® E), 6 cm = 12p, 8 cm = 15p, 10 cm = 17p, 12 cm = 21p (Hartmann)

Cotton Conforming Bandage, BP 1988
Cotton fabric, plain weave, treated to impart some elasticity to warp and weft. 3.5 m (all): type A, 5 cm = 63p, 7.5 cm = 77p, 10 cm = 96p, 15 cm = £1.30 (S&N Hlth— *Easifix Crinx*®)

Knitted Polyamide and Cellulose Contour Bandage, BP 1988
Fabric, knitted warp of polyamide filament, weft of cotton or viscose, fast edges, one continuous length. 4 m stretched (all):
K-Band®, 5 cm = 19p, 7 cm = 24p, 10 cm = 26p, 15 cm = 46p (Urgo)
Knit-Band®, 5 cm = 10p, 7 cm = 15p, 10 cm = 17p, 15 cm = 30p (CliniMed)
Knit Fix®, 5 cm = 12p, 7 cm = 17p, 10 cm = 17p, 15 cm = 33p (Steraid)

Polyamide and Cellulose Contour Bandage, BP 1988
(formerly Nylon and Viscose Stretch Bandage)
Fabric, plain weave, warp of polyamide filament, weft of cotton or viscose, fast edges, one continuous length, 4 m stretched (all):
Acti-Wrap®, cohesive, latex-free, 6 cm = 43p, 8 cm = 62p, 10 cm = 74p (Activa)
Easifix®, 5 cm = 33p, 7.5 cm = 40p, 10 cm = 47p, 15 cm = 80p (S&N Hlth)
Kontour®, cohesive, 5 cm = 28p, 7.5 cm = 35p, 10 cm = 40p, 15 cm = 66p (Easigrip)
Slinky®, 5 cm = 39p, 7.5 cm = 55p, 10 cm = 66p, 15 cm = 95p (Medlock)
Stayform®, 5 cm = 29p, 7.5 cm = 36p, 10 cm = 40p, 15 cm = 68p (Robinsons)

A8.8.3 Tubular bandages and garments

Tubular bandages are available in different forms, according to the function required of them. Some are used under orthopaedic casts and some are suitable for protecting areas to which creams or ointments (other than those containing potent corticosteroids) have been applied. The conformability of the elasticated versions makes them particularly suitable for retaining dressings on difficult parts of the body or for soft tissue injury, but their use as the only means of applying pressure to an oedematous limb or to a varicose ulcer is not appropriate, since the pressure they exert is inadequate.

Compression hosiery (section A8.9.1) reduces the recurrence of venous leg ulcers and should be considered after wound healing.

Silk clothing is available as an alternative to elasticated viscose stockinette garments, for use in the management of severe eczema and allergic skin conditions (see below).

◄Elasticated

Elasticated Surgical Tubular Stockinette, Foam padded
(Drug Tariff specification 25). Fabric as for Elasticated Tubular Bandage with polyurethane foam lining. Heel, elbow, knee, small = £2.68, medium = £2.83, large = £3.09; sacral,, medium, and large (all) = £13.82 (Medlock—*Tubipad*®)
Uses relief of pressure and elimination of friction in relevant area; porosity of foam lining allows normal water loss from skin surface

Elasticated Tubular Bandage, BP 1993
(formerly Elasticated Surgical Tubular Stockinette). Knitted fabric, elasticated threads of rubber-cored polyamide or polyester with cotton or cotton and viscose yarn, tubular. Lengths 50 cm and 1 m, widths 6.25 cm, 6.75 cm, 7.5 cm, 8.75 cm, 10 cm, 12 cm; Synergy—*Comfigrip*®; Easigrip—*EasiGRIP*®; Sallis—*Eesiban*®; Sigma—*Sigma ETB*®; Medlock—*Tubigrip*®. Where no size stated by prescriber the 50 cm length should be supplied and width endorsed

Elasticated Viscose Stockinette

(Drug Tariff specification 46). Lightweight plain-knitted elasticated tubular bandage.

Acti-Fast®, 3.5 cm red line (small limb), length 1 m = 62p; 5 cm green line (medium limb), length 1 m = 65p, 3 m = £1.90, 5 m = £3.30; 7.5 cm blue line (large limb), length 1 m = 90p, 3 m = £2.50, 5 m = £4.40; 10.75 cm yellow line (child trunk), length 1 m = £1.45, 3 m = £4.10, 5 m = £7.10; 17.5 cm beige line (adult trunk), length 1 m = £2.15 (Activa)

CliniFast®, 3.5 cm red line (small limb), length 1 m = 56p; 5 cm green line (medium limb), length 1 m = 58p, 3 m = £1.62, 5 m = £2.81; 7.5 cm blue line (large limb), length 1 m = 77p, 3 m = £2.13, 5 m = £3.74; 10.75 cm yellow line (child trunk), length 1 m = £1.20, 3 m = £3.49, 5 m = £6.04; 17.5 cm beige line (adult trunk), length 1 m = £1.83; vest (long-sleeved), 6–24 months = £7.13, 2–5 years = £9.50, 5–8 years = £10.69, 8–11 years = £11.88, 11–14 years = £11.88, adult, small, = £12.75, medium = £14.54, large = £16.58; vest (short-sleeved), adult, small = £12.50, medium = £14.25, large = £16.25; tights (pair) 6–24 months = £7.13; leggings (pair) 2–5 years = £9.50, 5–8 years = £10.69, 8–11 years = £11.88, 11–14 years = £11.88, adult, small, = £12.75, medium = £14.54, large = £16.58; cycle shorts, adult, small = £12.50, medium = £14.25, large = £16.25; socks (pair) up to 8 years = £2.97, 8–14 years = £2.97; mittens (pair) up to 24 months = £2.97, 2–8 years = £2.97, 8–14 years = £2.97; clava 6 months–5 years = £5.85, 5–14 years = £6.75 (Clinisupplies)

Comfifast®, 3.5 cm red line (small limb), length 1 m = 59p; 5 cm green line (medium limb), length 1 m = 61p, 3 m = £1.67, 5 m = £2.86; 7.5 cm blue line (large limb), length 1 m = 81p, 3 m = £2.19, 5 m = £3.80; 10.75 cm yellow line (child trunk), length 1 m = £1.26, 3 m = £3.54, 5 m = £6.09; 17.5 cm beige line (adult trunk), length 1 m = £1.88 (Synergy)

Comfifast® Easy Wrap, vest (long-sleeved), 6–24 months = £8.08, 2–5 years = £10.77, 5–8 years = £12.12, 8–11 years = £13.46, 11–14 years = £13.46, adult, small = £15.30, medium = £17.44, large = 19.89; tights (pair) 6–24 months = £8.08; leggings (pair) 2–5 years = £10.77, 5–8 years = £12.12, 8–11 years = £13.46, 11–14 years = £13.46, adult, small = £15.30, medium = £17.44, large = £19.89; socks (pair) up to 8 years = £3.37, 8–14 = £3.37; mittens (pair) up to 24 months = £3.37, 2–8 years = £3.37, 8–14 years = £3.37; clava, 6 months–5 years = £6.63, 5–14 years = £7.65 (Synergy)

Coverflex®, 3.5 cm red line (small limb), length 1 m = 75p; 5 cm green line (medium limb), length 1 m = 78p, 3 m = £2.28, 5 m = £3.94; 7.5 cm blue line (large limb), length 1 m = £1.09, 3 m = £2.60, 5 m = £ 5.14; 10.75 cm yellow line (child trunk), length 1 m = £1.71, 3 m = £4.93, 5 m = £8.67; 17.5 cm beige line (adult trunk), length 1 m = £2.28 (Hartmann)

Easifast®, 3.5 cm red line (small limb), length 1 m = 65p; 5 cm green line (medium limb), length 1 m = 69p, 3 m = £1.95, 5 m = £3.40; 7.5 cm blue line (large limb), length 1 m = 94p, 3 m = £2.60, 5 m = £4.50; 10.75 cm yellow line (child trunk), length 1 m = £1.50, 3 m = £4.25, 5 m = £7.20; 17.5 cm beige line (adult trunk), length 1 m = £1.90 (Easigrip)

Skinnies®, clava 6 months–5 years = £6.62, 5–14 years = £7.60; vest (long-sleeved) 6–24 months = £10.30, 2–5 years = £13.50, 5–8 years = £15.25, 8–11 years or 11–14 years = £16.90, adult (small) = £20.90, (medium) = £22.80, (large) = £24.70; body-suit 0–3 months or 3–6 months = £15.90; leggings (pair) 6–24 months = £10.30, 2–5 years = £13.50, 5–8 years = £15.25, 8–11 years or 11–14 years = £16.90, adult (small) = £20.90, (medium) = £22.80, (large) = £24.70; socks (pair) 6 months–8 years or 8–14 years = £4.20; mittens 0–24 months, 2–8 years, or 8–14 years = £3.80; gloves child (small) = £5.20, (medium or large) = £5.25, adult (small) = £5.20, (medium or large) = £5.25. (Skinnies)

Tubifast®, 3.5 cm red line (small limb), length 1 m = 85p; 5 cm green line (medium limb), length 1 m = 92p, 3 m = £2.62, 5 m = £4.49; 7.5 cm blue line (large limb), length 1 m = £1.23, 3 m = £3.45, 5 m = £6.02; 10.75 cm yellow line (child trunk), length 1 m = £1.07, 3 m = £5.02, 5 m = £9.00; 20 cm purple line (large adult trunk), length 1 m = £3.18, 5 m = £15.57; vest (long-sleeved) 6–24 months = £10.68, 2–5 years = £14.23, 5–8 years = £16.01, 8–11 years = £17.79, 11–14 years = £17.79; tights (pair) 6–24 months = £10.68; leggings (pair) 2–5 years = £14.23, 5–8 years = £16.01, 8–11 years = £17.79, 11–14 years = £17.79; socks (pair) = £4.45; gloves (small, medium or large adult, medium or large child) = £5.46 (Medlock)

◢ Non-elasticated
Cotton Stockinette, Bleached, BP 1988

Knitted fabric, cotton yarn, tubular length, 1 m (all), 2.5 cm = 33p; 5 cm = 51p; 7.5 cm = 62p; 6 m × 10 cm = £4.23 (J&J, Medlock)

Uses 1 m lengths, basis (with wadding) for Plaster of Paris bandages etc.; 6 m length, compression bandage

Ribbed Cotton and Viscose Surgical Tubular Stockinette, BP 1988

Knitted fabric of 1:1 ribbed structure, singles yarn spun from blend of two-thirds cotton and one-third viscose fibres, tubular. Length 5 m (all):

type A (lightweight): arm/leg (child), arm (adult) 5 cm = £2.40; arm (OS adult), leg (adult) 7.5 cm = £3.15; leg (OS adult) 10 cm = £4.18; trunk (child) 15 cm = £6.02; trunk (adult) 20 cm = £6.95; trunk (OS adult) 25 cm = £8.31 (Mölnlycke)

type B (heavyweight): sizes as for type A, net price £2.30–£7.97 (Sallis—*Eesiban*®)

Drug Tariff specifies various combinations of sizes to provide sufficient material for part or full body coverage

Uses protective dressings with tar-based and other non-steroid ointments

◢ Silk Clothing

Knitted, medical grade silk clothing can be used as an adjunct to normal treatment for severe eczema and allergic skin conditions. When used in combination with medical creams and ointments, care should be taken to ensure that the medication is fully absorbed into the skin before the silk clothing is worn; silk garments are not suitable for use in direct contact with emollients used in 'wet wrapping techniques'.

DermaSilk® (Espere)

Knitted silk fabric, hypoallergenic, sericin-free, *body suit*, child up to 6 months (height 68 cm) = £35.65, 6–9 months (height 74 cm) = £36.67, 12–18 months (height 86 cm) = £36.69, 2–3 years (height 98 cm) = £38.71, 3–4 years (height 110 cm) = £39.73; *Facial mask*, child 6–12 months = £15.30, 1–6 years = £15.30; *Gloves*, adult (small, medium or large) = £19.33, child 3–4 years = £13.77, 5–9 years = £13.77; *Leggings*, child up to 6 months (height 68 cm) = £25.45, 6–9 months (height 74 cm) = £26.47, 12–18 months (height 86 cm) = £27.49, 2–3 years (height 98 cm) = £28.51, 3–4 years (height 110 cm) = £29.53; *Pyjamas*, child 3–4 years (height 110 cm) = £66.25, 5–6 years (height 120 cm) = £70.33, 7–8 years (height 135 cm) = £73.39, 10–12 years (height 150 cm) = £76.45; *Sleeves (tubular)* one size = £25.45; *Undersocks, (heel-less)*, 2 pairs standard or longer length = £22.95; *Undersocks*, adult shoe-size 5½–6½, 7–8½, 9–10½, 11–13, child shoe-size 3–8, 9–1, 2–5, 2 pairs = £17.45

A8.8.4 Support bandages

Light support bandages, which include the various forms of crepe bandage, are used in the prevention of oedema; they are also used to provide support for mild sprains and joints but their effectiveness has not been proven for this purpose. Since they have limited extensibility, they are able to provide light support without exerting undue pressure. For a warning against injudicious compression see section A8.8.7.

Crepe Bandage, BP 1988

Fabric, plain weave, warp of wool threads and crepe-twisted cotton threads, weft of cotton threads; stretch bandage. 4.5 m stretched (all): 5 cm = 90p; 7.5 cm = £1.26; 10 cm = £1.65; 15 cm = £2.39 (most suppliers)

Cotton Crepe Bandage

Light support bandage, 4.5 m stretched (all): 5 cm = 48p; 7.5 cm = 67p; 10 cm = 87p; 15 cm = £1.27 (Steraid—*Hospicrepe*® 239)

Cotton Crepe Bandage, BP 1988

Fabric, plain weave, warp of crepe-twisted cotton threads, weft of cotton and/or viscose threads; stretch bandage. 4.5 m stretched (both): 7.5 cm = £2.81; 10 cm = £3.62; other sizes 〔NHS〕 (most suppliers)

Cotton, Polyamide and Elastane Bandage

Fabric, cotton, polyamide, and elastane; light support bandage (Type 2), 4.5 m stretched (all): 5 cm = 54p, 7.5 cm = 73p, 10 cm = 91p, 15 cm = £1.12 (Neomedic—*Neosport*®); 5 cm = 64p, 7.5 cm = 91p, 10 cm = £1.16, 15 cm = £1.67 (BSN Medical—*Softcrepe*®); 10 cm = £1.10 (Mölnlycke—*Setocrepe*®); 10 cm = £1.24, latex-free = £1.31 (S&N Hlth.—*Profore*® #2)

Cotton Stretch Bandage, BP 1988

Fabric, plain weave, warp of crepe-twisted cotton threads, weft of cotton threads; stretch bandage, lighter than cotton crepe, 4.5 m stretched (all):

Hospicrepe® 233, 5 cm = 52p; 7.5 cm = 72p; 10 cm = 96p; 15 cm = £1.36 (Steraid)

PremierBand®, 5 cm = 45p, 7.5 cm = 63p, 10 cm = 79p, 15 cm = £1.18 (Shermond)

Cotton Suspensory Bandage

(Drug Tariff). Type 1: cotton net bag with draw tapes and webbing waistband; small, medium, and large (all) = £1.55, extra large = £1.65. Type 2: cotton net bag with elastic edge and webbing waistband; small = £1.72, medium = £1.77, large = £1.83, extra large = £1.91. Type 3: cotton net bag with elastic edge and webbing waistband with elastic insertion; small, medium, and large (all) = £1.86; extra large = £1.92. Type supplied to be endorsed

Knitted Elastomer and Viscose Bandage

Knitted fabric, viscose and elastomer yarn.

Type 2 (light support bandage)

CliniLite®, 4.5 m (all), 5 cm = 44p, 7.5 cm = 61p, 10 cm = 80p, 15 cm = £1.16 (Clinisupplies)

K-Lite®, 4.5 m stretched, 5 cm = 51p, 7 cm = 71p, 10 cm = 93p, 15 cm = £1.34; 5.2 m stretched, 10 cm = £1.06 (Urgo)

Knit-Firm®, 4.5 m stretched, 5 cm = 36p, 7 cm = 51p, 10 cm = 66p, 15 cm = 96p (Steraid)

Type 3a (light compression bandage):

CliniPlus®, 8.7 m × 10 cm = £1.80 (Clinisupplies)

Elset®, 6 m stretched, 10 cm = £2.39, 15 cm = £2.59; 8 m stretched, 10 cm = £3.06; 12 m stretched, 15 cm = £5.13 (Mölnlycke)

K-Plus®, 8.7 m stretched, 10 cm = £2.08 (Urgo)

K-Plus® Long, 10.25 m stretched, 10 cm = £2.41 (Urgo)

Profore® #3, 8.7 m stretched, 10 cm = £3.60, latex-free = £3.91 (S&N Hlth.)

L3, 8.6 m stretched, 10 cm = £2.04 (S&N Hlth.)

A8.8.5 Adhesive bandages

Elastic adhesive bandages are used to provide compression in the treatment of varicose veins and for the support of injured joints; they should no longer be used for the support of fractured ribs and clavicles. They have also been used with **zinc paste bandage** in the treatment of venous ulcers, but they can cause skin reactions in susceptible patients and may not produce sufficient pressures for healing (significantly lower than those provided by other compression bandages).

Elastic Adhesive Bandage, BP 1993

Woven fabric, elastic in warp (crepe-twisted cotton threads), weft of cotton and/or viscose threads spread with adhesive mass containing zinc oxide. 4.5 m stretched (all): 5 cm = £3.31; 7.5 cm = £4.80; 10 cm = £6.38 (Robinsons—

Flexoplast®; S&N Hlth—*Elastoplast*® Bandage). 7.5 cm width supplied when size not stated

A8.8.6 Cohesive bandages

Cohesive bandages adhere to themselves, but not to the skin, and are useful for providing support for sports use where ordinary stretch bandages might become displaced and adhesive bandages are inappropriate. Care is needed in their application, however, since the loss of ability for movement between turns of the bandage to equalise local areas of high tension carries the potential for creating a tourniquet effect. They should not be used if arterial disease is suspected.

◢Cohesive extensible bandages

These elastic bandages adhere to themselves and not to skin; this prevents slipping during use.
Uses: support of sprained joints; outer layer of multi-layer compression bandaging

Coban® (3M)
6 m (stretched), 10 cm = £2.76; other sizes 〔NHS〕 4.5 m stretched (all): 2.5 cm = £1.29; 5 cm = £1.81; 7.5 cm = £2.74; 10 cm = £3.61; 15 cm = £5.33

K-Press® (Urgo)
6.5 m × 10 cm (0, short) = £2.76, 7.5 m × 10 cm (18–25 cm ankle circumference) = £3.22, 10.5 m × 10 cm (25–32 cm ankle circumference) = £3.53

Profore® #4 (S&N Hlth.)
2.5 m (unstretched) = £2.97, latex-free = £3.23

Ultra Fast® (Robinsons)
6.3 m (stretched), 10 cm = £2.59

A8.8.7 Compression bandages

High compression products are used to provide the high compression needed for the management of gross varices, post-thrombotic venous insufficiency, venous leg ulcers, and gross oedema in average-sized limbs. Their use calls for an expert knowledge of the elastic properties of the products and experience in the technique of providing careful graduated compression. Incorrect application can lead to uneven and inadequate pressures or to hazardous levels of pressure. In particular, injudicious use of compression in limbs with arterial disease has been reported to cause severe skin and tissue necrosis (in some instances calling for amputation). Doppler testing is required before treatment with compression. Oral pentoxifylline (BNF section 2.6.4) can be used as adjunct therapy if a chronic venous leg ulcer does not respond to compression bandaging [unlicensed indication].

◢High compression bandages
PEC High Compression Bandage

Polyamide, elastane, and cotton compression (high) extensible bandage, 3.5 m unstretched (both): 7.5 cm = £2.51; 10 cm = £3.25 (Mölnlycke—*Setopress*®)

VEC High Compression Bandage

Viscose, elastane, and cotton compression (high) extensible bandage, 3 m unstretched (both): 7.5 cm = £2.53; 10 cm = £3.25 (S&N—*Tensopress*®)

High Compression Bandage

Cotton, viscose, nylon, and Lycra® extensible bandage, 3 m (unstretched), 10 cm = £3.33 (ConvaTec— *SurePress*®);

3 m (unstretched), 10 cm = £2.64 (Urgo—*K-ThreeC*®); 3.5 m (unstretched), 10 cm = £1.82 (Advancis—*Adva-Co*®)

ProGuide® #2 (S&N Hlth.)
Woven, elastomer, cohesive, extensible, compression bandage, 3 m (unstretched), 10 cm (red) = £5.37, 10 cm (yellow) = £5.85, 10 cm (green) = £6.34

◼ **Short stretch compression bandage**
Short stretch bandages help to reduce oedema and promote healing of venous leg ulcers. They are also used to reduce swelling associated with lymphoedema. They are applied at full stretch over padding (*see* Sub-compression Wadding Bandage below) which protects areas of high pressure and sites at high risk of pressure damage.

Actiban® (Activa)
All 5 m, 8 cm = £3.08; 10 cm = £3.31; 12 cm = £4.02

Actico® (Activa)
Cohesive, all 6 m, 4 cm = £2.19, 6 cm = £2.57, 8 cm = £2.95, 10 cm = £3.07, 12 cm = £3.91

Comprilan® (BSN Medical)
All 5 m, 6 cm = £2.52; 8 cm = £2.96; 10 cm = £3.18; 12 cm = £3.87

Rosidal K® (Activa)
All 5 m, 4cm = £1.73, 6cm = £2.42, 8 cm = £2.89, 10 cm = £3.15, 12 cm = £3.83; 10m x 10cm = £5.49

Silkolan® (Urgo)
All 5 m, 8 cm = £3.00; 10 cm = £3.39

◼ **Sub-compression wadding bandage**
Advasoft® (Advancis)
3.5 m unstretched, 10 cm = 37p

Cellona® Undercast Padding (Activa)
2.75 m unstretched (all): 5 cm = 29p, 7.5 cm = 35p; 10 cm = 43p; 15 cm = 55p

Flexi-Ban® (Activa)
Padding, 3.5 m unstretched, 10cm = 46p

K-Soft® (Urgo)
3.5 m unstretched, 10 cm = 42p; 4.5 m unstretched, 10 cm = 52p

K-Tech® (Urgo)
5 m stretched, 10 cm (0, short) = £3.73, 6 m unstretched, 10 cm (18–25 cm ankle circumference) = £4.48, 7.3 m unstretched, 10 cm (25–32 cm ankle circumference) = £4.89

Ortho-Band Plus® (Steraid)
10 cm × 3.5 cm unstretched = 37p

Profore® #1 (S&N Hlth.)
Viscose fleece, 3.5 m unstretched, 10 cm = 64p, latex-free = 70p

ProGuide® #1 (S&N Hlth.)
Polyester and viscose fleece, 4 m unstretched, 10 cm = £1.49

Softexe® (Mölnlycke)
3.5 m unstretched, 10 cm = 58p

SurePress® (ConvaTec)
Absorbent padding, 3 m unstretched, 10 cm = 56p

Ultra Soft® (Robinsons)
Soft absorbent bandage, 3.5 m unstretched, 10 cm = 39p

Velband® (BSN Medical)
Absorbent padding, 4.5 m unstretched, 10 cm = 67p

A8.8.8 Multi-layer compression bandaging

Multi-layer compression bandaging systems are an alternative to High Compression Bandages (section A8.8.7) for the treatment of venous leg ulcers. Compression is achieved by the combined effects of two or three extensible bandages applied over a layer of orthopaedic wadding and a wound contact dressing.

◼ **Four layer systems**
K-Four® (Urgo)
K-Four® Wound Dressing (*Paratex*—see Knitted Viscose Primary Dressing, p. 35); *K-Four® # 1* (*K-Soft*®—see Sub-compression Wadding Bandage, above); *K-Four® # 2* (*K-Lite*®—see Knitted Elastomer and Viscose Bandage, p. 50); *K-Four® # 3* (*K-Plus*®—see Knitted Elastomer and Viscose Bandage, p. 50); *K-Three C*®—see High compression bandages, p. 50; *K-Four® # 4* (*Ko-Flex*®), 6 m (stretched), 10 cm = £2.76; 7 m (stretched), 10 cm = £3.16
Multi-layer compression bandaging kit, four layer system, for ankle circumference up to 18 cm = £6.93, 18–25 cm = £6.51, 25–30 cm = £6.64, above 30 cm = £9.05; *reduced compression*, 18 cm+ = £4.43

Profore® (S&N Hlth.)
Profore® wound contact layer (see Knitted Viscose Primary Dressing, p. 35); *Profore® #1* (see Sub-compression Wadding Bandage, above); *Profore® #2* (see Cotton, Polyamide and Elastane Bandage, p. 50); *Profore® #3* (see Knitted Elastomer and Viscose Bandage, p. 50); *Profore® #4* (see Cohesive bandages, p. 50); *Profore® Plus* 3 m (unstretched), 10 cm = £3.37, latex-free = £3.60
Multi-layer compression bandaging kit, four layer system, for ankle circumference up to 18 cm = £9.32, 18–25 cm = £8.68, 25–30 cm = £7.21, above 30 cm = £10.79, latex-free, 18–25 cm = £9.28; *Profore Lite®* above 18 cm = £5.01, latex-free = £5.45

System 4® (Mölnlycke)
System 4® #1 (*Softexe*®—see Sub-compression Wadding Bandage, above); *System 4® #2* (*Setocrepe*®—see Cotton, Polyamide and Elastane Bandage, p. 50); *System 4® #3* (*Elset*®—see Knitted Elastomer and Viscose Bandage, p. 50); *System 4® #4* (*Coban*®—see Cohesive Bandages, p. 50)
Multi-layer compression bandaging kit, four layer system, for ankle circumference 18–25 cm = £7.51

Ultra Four® (Robinsons)
Ultra Four® #1 (*Ultra Soft*®—see Sub-compression Wadding Bandage, above); *Ultra Four® #2* (*Ultra Lite*®) 10 cm × 4.5 cm (stretched) = 85p; *Ultra Four® #3* (*Ultra Plus*®) 10 cm × 0.7 cm (stretched) = £1.09; *Ultra Four® #4* (*Ultra Fast*®— see Cohesive Bandages, p. 50)
Multi-layer compression bandaging kit, four layer system, for ankle circumference up to 18 cm = £6.41, 18–25 cm = £5.67; *Ultra Four® RC* (reduced compression) 18–25 cm = £4.14

◼ **Two layer systems**
Coban® (3M)
Multi-layer compression bandaging kit, two layer system (latex-free, foam bandage and cohesive compression bandage), one size = £8.08

K-Two® (Urgo)
K-Tech® (see Sub-compression Wadding Bandages, above); *K-Press®* (see Cohesive Bandages, p. 50)
Multi-layer compression bandaging kit, two layer system, ankle circumference 18–25 cm (short) = £6.50, ankle circumference 18–25 cm = £7.70, ankle circumference 25–32 cm = £8.41

K-Two® Start, *Urgotul®* Start (see Soft polymer dressings, p. 37); *K-Tech®* (see Sub-compression Wadding Bandages, p. 51); *K-Press®* (see Cohesive Bandages, p. 50)

Multi-layer compression bandaging kit, two-layer system, for ankle circumference 18–25cm = £9.68; 25–32cm = £10.33

ProGuide® (S&N Hlth.)

ProGuide® wound contact layer (see Soft polymer dressings, p. 38); *ProGuide®* #1 (see Sub-compression Wadding Bandage, p. 51); *ProGuide®* #2 (see High Compression Bandages, p. 51)

Multi-layer compression bandaging kit, two layer system, for ankle circumference 18–22 cm (red) = £8.98; 22–28 cm (yellow) = £9.48; 28–32 cm (green) = £9.96

A8.8.9 Medicated bandages

Zinc Paste Bandage has been used with compression bandaging for the treatment of venous leg ulcers. However, paste bandages are associated with hypersensitivity reactions and should be used with caution.

Zinc paste bandages are also used with **coal tar** or **ichthammol** in chronic lichenified skin conditions such as chronic eczema (ichthammol often being preferred since its action is considered to be milder). They are also used with **calamine** in milder eczematous skin conditions.

Zinc Paste Bandage, BP 1993

Cotton fabric, plain weave, impregnated with suitable paste containing zinc oxide; requires additional bandaging, 6 m × 7.5 cm = £3.23 (S&N Hlth.—*Viscopaste PB7®* (10%), *excipients: include* cetostearyl alcohol, hydroxybenzoates)

Zinc Paste and Calamine Bandage

(Drug Tariff specification 5). Cotton fabric, plain weave, impregnated with suitable paste containing calamine and zinc oxide; requires additional bandaging. 6 m × 7.5 cm = £3.33 (Mölnlycke—*Calaband®*)

Zinc Paste and Ichthammol Bandage, BP 1993

Cotton fabric, plain weave, impregnated with suitable paste containing zinc oxide and ichthammol; requires additional bandaging, 6 m × 7.5 cm = £3.31 S&N Hlth.—*Ichthopaste®* (6/2%), *excipients: include* cetostearyl alcohol

Uses see BNF section 13.5

Steripaste® (Mölnlycke)

Cotton fabric, selvedge weave impregnated with paste containing zinc oxide (requires additional bandaging), 6 m × 7.5 cm = £3.24

Excipients include polysorbate 80

◀**Medicated stocking**

Zipzoc® (S&N Hlth.)

Sterile rayon stocking impregnated with ointment containing zinc oxide 20%. 4-pouch carton = £12.52; 10-pouch carton = £31.30

Note Can be used under appropriate compression bandages or hosiery in chronic venous insufficiency

A8.9 Compression hosiery and garments

Compression (elastic) hosiery is used to treat conditions associated with chronic venous insufficiency, to prevent recurrence of thrombosis, or to reduce the risk of further venous ulceration after treatment with compression bandaging (section A8.8.7). Doppler testing to confirm arterial sufficiency is required before recommending the use of compression hosiery.

Before elastic hosiery can be dispensed, the quantity (single or pair), article (including accessories), and compression class must be specified by the prescriber. There are different compression values for graduated compression hosiery and lymphoedema garments (see table below). All dispensed elastic hosiery articles must state on the packaging that they conform with Drug Tariff technical specification No. 40, for further details see Drug Tariff.

Note Graduated compression tights are 📋.

Compression values for hosiery and lymphoedema garments		
Compression class	Compression hosiery (British standard)	Lymphoedema garments (European classification)
Class 1	14–17 mmHg	18–21 mmHg
Class 2	18–24 mmHg	23–32 mmHg
Class 3	25–35 mmHg	34–46 mmHg
Class 4	Not available	49–70 mmHg
Class 4 super	Not available	60–90 mmHg

A8.9.1 Graduated compression hosiery

Class 1 Light Support

Hosiery, compression at ankle 14–17 mmHg, thigh length or below knee with knitted in heel. 1 pair, circular knit (standard), thigh length = £7.44, below knee = £6.80, (made-to-measure), thigh length = £36.95, below knee = £23.12; lightweight elastic net (made-to-measure), thigh length = £19.93, below knee = £15.55

Uses superficial or early varices, varicosis during pregnancy

Class 2 Medium Support

Hosiery, compression at ankle 18–24 mmHg, thigh length or below knee with knitted in heel. 1 pair, circular knit (standard), thigh length = £11.06, below knee = £9.94, (made-to-measure), thigh length = £36.95, below knee = £23.12; net (made-to-measure), thigh length = £19.93, below knee = £15.55; flat bed (made-to-measure, only with closed heel and open toe), thigh length = £36.95, below knee = £23.12

Uses varices of medium severity, ulcer treatment and prophylaxis, mild oedema, varicosis during pregnancy

Class 3 Strong Support

Hosiery, compression at ankle 25–35 mmHg, thigh length or below knee with open or knitted in heel. 1 pair, circular knit (standard), thigh length = £13.11, below knee = £11.27, (made-to-measure) thigh length = £36.95, below knee = £23.12; flat bed (made-to-measure, only with open heel and open toe), thigh length = £36.95, below knee = £23.12

Uses gross varices, post thrombotic venous insufficiency, gross oedema, ulcer treatment and prophylaxis

◀**Accessories**

In addition to the product listed below, accessories such as application aids for hosiery are available, see Drug Tariff for details

Suspender

Suspender, for thigh stockings = 65p, belt (specification 13), = £4.96, fitted (additional price) = 62p

◢Anklets
Class 2 Medium Support
Anklets, compression 18–24 mmHg, circular knit (standard and made-to-measure), 1 pair = £6.51; flat bed (standard and made-to-measure) = £13.53; net (made-to-measure) = £12.80

Class 3 Strong Support
Anklets, compression 25–35 mmHg, circular knit (standard and made-to-measure), 1 pair = £9.09; flat bed (standard) = £9.09, (made-to-measure) = £13.53

◢Knee caps
Class 2 Medium Support
Kneecaps, compression 18–24 mmHg, circular knit (standard and made-to-measure), 1 pair = £6.51; flat bed (standard and made-to-measure) = £13.53; net (made-to-measure) = £10.63

Class 3 Strong Support
Kneecaps, compression 25–35 mmHg, circular knit (standard and made-to-measure), 1 pair = £8.68; flat bed (standard) = £8.68, (made-to-measure) = £13.53

A8.9.2 Lymphoedema garments

Lymphoedema compression garments are used to maintain limb shape and prevent additional fluid retention.

In addition to the products listed below, made-to-measure garments up to compression 90 mmHg and accessories also available; see Drug Tariff for details. There are different compression values for lymphoedema garments and graduated compression hosiery, see table, p. 52

Low Compression
Armsleeves (with grip top), compression 12–16 mmHg, small, medium, and large sizes all available short or long, 1 pair = £16.70

Class 1 Light support
Hosiery and armsleeves, compression 18–21 mmHg, small, medium, large, and extra large (hosiery only) sizes all available standard length (some available petite), 1 pair below knee closed toe (no top band) = £25.50, thigh closed toe (with top band) = £49.00; 1 piece armsleeve (no top band) = £13.50, armsleeve (with top band) = £18.00, combined armsleeve (no top band) = £24.50, combined armsleeve (with top band) = £29.00

Armsleeves (with grip top), compression 18–22 mmHg, small, medium, and large sizes all available short or long, 1 pair = £16.70

Class 2 Medium support
Hosiery and armsleeves, compression 23–32 mmHg, small, medium, large, and extra large (hosiery only) sizes all available standard length (some available petite), 1 pair below knee closed or open toe (no top band) = £25.50, thigh closed or open toe (with top band) = £49.00; 1 piece armsleeve (no top band) = £14.50, armsleeve (with top band) = £19.00, combined armsleeve (no top band) = £25.50, combined armsleeve (with top band) = £30.00

Class 3 Strong support
Hosiery, compression 34–46 mmHg, small, medium, large, and extra large sizes all available standard length (some available petite), 1 pair below knee open toe (no top band) = £28.00, thigh open toe (with top band) = £51.00

Index

Proprietary (trade) names and names of organisms are printed in *italic* type.

A

Abbreviations, *inside back cover*
    Latin, *inside back cover*
Absorbent cotton, bandages, dressings, gauze, 35, 45, 46
Actiban, 51
Actico, 51
Acticoat products, 43
Acti-Fast, 49
ActiFormCool, 36
Actilite, 42
Actisorb Silver, 43
Activated charcoal dressings, 41
ActivHeal products
    alginate, 40
    film dressing, 36
    foam, 39, 40
    hydrocolloid, 38
    hydrogel, 36
Activon products, 42
Acti-Wrap, 48
Adhesive
    dressings, 47
    films, 36
Adva-Co, 50
Advadraw products, 41
Advasil, 44
Advasoft, 51
Advazorb products, 39, 40
Adverse reactions, 2
Airstrip, 47
Alginate dressings, 40, 41, 42, 43
Algisite products, 40, 43
Algivon, 42
Algosteril products, 40
Alione, 38
Alldress, 37
Allevyn products, 37, 39, 40, 43
Almond oil ear drops, 17
Anaesthetics, local, 13
Analgesics, 11
Anthelmintics, 18
Antimicrobial dressings, 41
Aquacel products, 39, 43
Aquaflo, 36
Aquaform, 36
Aqueous cream, 21
Arachis oil
    enema, 9
    presence of, 1
    skin, 21
Askina products
    charcoal, 41
    film dressing, 35, 36
    foam, 40
    hydrocolloid, 38
    hydrogel, 36
Aspartame, presence of, 1
Aspirin, 11
Atrauman products, 35, 43
Avance products, 43

B

Bactigras, 44
Balneum bath oil, 22
Bandages, 48–52
Barrier preparations, 23
Biatain products, 39, 40
    silver with, 43
Bioclusive, 36
Biotrol products, 45
Bisacodyl, 7
Blenderm, 47
Blisterfilm, 36
Blood glucose monitoring, 29
Boils, 24

C

Cadesorb, 44
Cadexomer–iodine, 42
Calaband, 26, 52
Calamine, 24
Calcium alginate dressings, 40, 42, 43
Capillary-action dressings, 41
CarboFLEX, 41
Carbopad VC, 41
Catheter patency solutions, 27
Catheters, urethral, 27
Cavi-Care, 40
Cellona, 51
Central Gard, 37
Cerdak products, 41
Cetraben
    cream, 21
    emollient bath additive, 22
Charcoal, activated dressings, 41, 43
Children, prescribing for, 1
Chlorhexidine
    catheter maintenance solution, 27
    dressing, gauze, 44
    skin disinfection, 25
Choline salicylate, 16
    dental gel, 17
Cica-Care, 44
Ciltech, 44
Cleansing, skin, 25
CliniFast, 49
CliniLite, 50
CliniPlus, 50
Clinipore, 47
Clinisorb, 41
Clotrimazole, 24
Coban, 50, 51
Co-danthramer, 7
Co-danthrusate, 7
Colloid dressings, 38, 43
Colostomy, 28
Comfeel products, 38
Comfifast products, 49
Comfigrip, 48
Compression
    bandages, 50
    hosiery, graduated, 52

Comprilan, 51
Constipation, 6
Contraceptive devices
    caps (pessaries), 31
    diaphragms, 31
    intra-uterine, 30
    spermicidal, 31
Controlled drugs, independent prescribing, 5
Coolie, 36
Copa products, 39, 40
Cosmopor E, 35
Cotfil, 46
Cotton
    absorbent, 45
    gauze, 45
Coverflex, 49
Crotamiton, 19, 24
    cream, 24
    lotion, 24
Curasorb products, 40
Cuticell Classic, 35
Cutimed gel, 36
Cutimed Sorbact products, 44
Cutinova products, 39
Cutisorb LA, 35
C-View, 36

D

Dantron, 7
Denture stomatitis, 16
Dermalo, 22
Dermamist, 21
DermaSilk, 49
Dermasure products, 45
Dermatix products, 44
Diabetes
    appliances, 29
    diagnostic agents, 29
Dimeticone
    creams, 23
    head lice, 19
    spray, zinc oxide with, 23
Diprobase, 21
Diprobath, 22
Disinfection, skin, 25
Disposable gloves
    film, 10
    nitrile, 10
    polythene, 10
Docusate, 7, 8
Domette bandage, 48
Doublebase
    bath additive, 22
    gel, 21
    shower gel, 22
    wash gel, 22
Dressing packs, 46, 48
Dressings
    absorbent, 35
    advanced, 35
    antimicrobial, 41
    low adherence, 34
Dressit, 46
Drisorb, 45
Drug Tariff, information, 4
Dry mouth, treatment of, 17
DuoDERM products, 38

Yellowcard®

COMMISSION ON HUMAN MEDICINES

In Confidence

MHRA

SUSPECTED ADVERSE DRUG REACTIONS

If you suspect that an adverse reaction may be related to a drug, or a combination of drugs, you should complete this Yellow Card or complete a report on the website at www.yellowcard.gov.uk. For *intensively monitored medicines* (identified by ▼) report **all** suspected reactions (including any considered not to be serious). For *established drugs* and *herbal remedies* report **all serious** adverse reactions in adults; report **all serious and minor** adverse reactions in **children** (under 18 years). You do not have to be certain about causality: if in doubt, please report. Do not be put off reporting just because some details are not known. See BNF (page 11) or the MHRA website (www.yellowcard.gov.uk) for additional advice.

PATIENT DETAILS	Patient Initials: _____	Sex: M / F	Weight if known (kg): _____
Age (at time of reaction): _____	Identification (Your Practice / Hospital Ref.)*: _____		

SUSPECTED DRUG(S)

Give brand name of drug and batch number if known	Route	Dosage	Date started	Date stopped	Prescribed for

SUSPECTED REACTION(S)

Please describe the reaction(s) and any treatment given:

Outcome

- ☐ Recovered
- ☐ Recovering
- ☐ Continuing
- ☐ Other

Date reaction(s) started: _____   Date reaction(s) stopped: _____

Do you consider the reaction to be serious?   Yes / No

If *yes*, please indicate why the reaction is considered to be serious (please tick all that apply):

- ☐ Patient died due to reaction   ☐ Involved or prolonged inpatient hospitalisation
- ☐ Life threatening   ☐ Involved persistent or significant disability or incapacity
- ☐ Congenital abnormality   ☐ Medically significant; please give details:

* This is to enable you to identify the patient in any future correspondence concerning this report

Please attach additional pages if necessary

Please list other drugs taken in the last 3 months prior to the reaction (including self-medication & herbal remedies)

Was the patient on any other medication?   Yes / No   If *yes*, please give the following information if known:

Drug (Brand, if known)	Route	Dosage	Date started	Date stopped	Prescribed for

Additional relevant information e.g. medical history, test results, known allergies, rechallenge (if performed), suspected drug interactions. For congenital abnormalities please state all other drugs taken during pregnancy and the date of the last menstrual period.

REPORTER DETAILS	**CLINICIAN (if not the reporter)**
Name and Professional Address:	Name and Professional Address:
Post code: _____ Tel No: _____	Tel No: _____ Post code: _____
Speciality: _____	Speciality: _____
Signature: _____ Date: _____	If you would like information about other adverse reactions associated with the suspected drug, please tick this box ☐

If you report from an area served by a Yellow Card Centre (YCC), MHRA may ask the Centre to communicate with you, on its behalf, about your report. See BNF (page 11) for further details on YCCs. If you want only MHRA to contact you, please tick this box.   ☐

Send to **Medicines and Healthcare products Regulatory Agency, CHM FREEPOST, LONDON SW8 5BR**

Yellowcard®

COMMISSION ON HUMAN MEDICINES

In Confidence

MHRA

SUSPECTED ADVERSE DRUG REACTIONS

If you suspect that an adverse reaction may be related to a drug, or a combination of drugs, you should complete this Yellow Card or complete a report on the website at www.yellowcard.gov.uk. For *intensively monitored medicines* (identified by ▼) report **all** suspected reactions (including any considered not to be serious). For *established drugs* and *herbal remedies* report **all serious** adverse reactions in adults; report **all serious and minor** adverse reactions in **children** (under 18 years). You do not have to be certain about causality: if in doubt, please report. Do not be put off reporting just because some details are not known. See BNF (page 11) or the MHRA website (www.yellowcard.gov.uk) for additional advice.

PATIENT DETAILS   Patient Initials: _____   Sex: M / F   Weight if known (kg): _____

Age (at time of reaction): _____   Identification (Your Practice / Hospital Ref.)*: _____

SUSPECTED DRUG(S)

Give brand name of drug and batch number if known	Route	Dosage	Date started	Date stopped	Prescribed for

SUSPECTED REACTION(S)

Please describe the reaction(s) and any treatment given:

Date reaction(s) started: _____   Date reaction(s) stopped: _____

Do you consider the reaction to be serious?   Yes / No

If *yes*, please indicate why the reaction is considered to be serious (please tick all that apply):

Patient died due to reaction   ☐

Life threatening   ☐

Congenital abnormality   ☐

Involved or prolonged inpatient hospitalisation   ☐

Involved persistent or significant disability or incapacity   ☐

Medically significant; please give details: ☐

Outcome

Recovered   ☐

Recovering   ☐

Continuing   ☐

Other   ☐

☐ ☐

* This is to enable you to identify the patient in any future correspondence concerning this report

Please attach additional pages if necessary

Please list other drugs taken in the last 3 months prior to the reaction (including self-medication & herbal remedies)

Was the patient on any other medication?   Yes / No   *If yes,* please give the following information if known:

Drug (Brand, if known)	Route	Dosage	Date started	Date stopped	Prescribed for

Additional relevant information e.g. medical history, test results, known allergies, rechallenge (if performed), suspected drug interactions. For congenital abnormalities please state all other drugs taken during pregnancy and the date of the last menstrual period.

REPORTER DETAILS	**CLINICIAN (if not the reporter)**
Name and Professional Address:	Name and Professional Address:
Post code: _____ Tel No: _____	Post code: _____
Speciality: _____	Tel No: _____ Speciality: _____
Signature: _____ Date: _____	If you would like information about other adverse reactions associated with the suspected drug, please tick this box ☐

If you report from an area served by a Yellow Card Centre (YCC), MHRA may ask the Centre to communicate with you, on its behalf, about your report. See BNF (page 11) for further details on YCCs. If you want only MHRA to contact you, please tick this box. ☐

Send to **Medicines and Healthcare products Regulatory Agency, CHM FREEPOST, LONDON SW8 5BR**

Yellowcard

COMMISSION ON HUMAN MEDICINES

In Confidence

SUSPECTED ADVERSE DRUG REACTIONS

MHRA

If you suspect that an adverse reaction may be related to a drug, or a combination of drugs, you should complete this Yellow Card or complete a report on the website at www.yellowcard.gov.uk. For *intensively monitored medicines* (identified by ▼) report **all** suspected reactions (including any considered not to be serious). For *established drugs* and *herbal remedies* report **all serious** adverse reactions in adults; report **all serious and minor** adverse reactions in **children** (under 18 years). You do not have to be certain about causality: if in doubt, please report. Do not be put off reporting just because some details are not known. See BNF (page 11) or the MHRA website (www.yellowcard.gov.uk) for additional advice.

PATIENT DETAILS Patient Initials: _____	Sex: M / F	Weight if known (kg): _____
Age (at time of reaction): _____	Identification (Your Practice / Hospital Ref.)*:	

SUSPECTED DRUG(S)

Give brand name of drug and batch number if known	Route	Dosage	Date started	Date stopped	Prescribed for
_____	_____	_____	_____	_____	_____
_____	_____	_____	_____	_____	_____

SUSPECTED REACTION(S)

Please describe the reaction(s) and any treatment given:

Outcome

Recovered ☐
Recovering ☐
Continuing ☐
Other ☐

Date reaction(s) started: _____ Date reaction(s) stopped: _____

Do you consider the reaction to be serious? Yes / No

If *yes*, please indicate why the reaction is considered to be serious (please tick all that apply):

Patient died due to reaction ☐	Involved or prolonged inpatient hospitalisation ☐
Life threatening ☐	Involved persistent or significant disability or incapacity ☐
Congenital abnormality ☐	Medically significant; please give details: ☐

* This is to enable you to identify the patient in any future correspondence concerning this report

Please attach additional pages if necessary

Please list other drugs taken in the last 3 months prior to the reaction (including self-medication & herbal remedies)

Was the patient on any other medication?   Yes / No   If *yes*, please give the following information if known:

Drug (Brand, if known)	Route	Dosage	Date started	Date stopped	Prescribed for

Additional relevant information e.g. medical history, test results, known allergies, rechallenge (if performed), suspected drug interactions. For congenital abnormalities please state all other drugs taken during pregnancy and the date of the last menstrual period.

REPORTER DETAILS
Name and Professional Address: _____

Post code: _____   Tel No: _____

Speciality: _____

Signature: _____   Date: _____

CLINICIAN (if not the reporter)
Name and Professional Address: _____

Post code: _____

Tel No: _____   Speciality: _____

If you would like information about other adverse reactions associated with the suspected drug, please tick this box   ☐

If you report from an area served by a Yellow Card Centre (YCC), MHRA may ask the Centre to communicate with you, on its behalf, about your report. See BNF (page 11) for further details on YCCs. If you want only MHRA to contact you, please tick this box.   ☐

Send to **Medicines and Healthcare products Regulatory Agency, CHM FREEPOST, LONDON SW8 5BR**

Yellowcard

COMMISSION ON
HUMAN MEDICINES

In Confidence

MHRA

SUSPECTED ADVERSE DRUG REACTIONS

If you suspect that an adverse reaction may be related to a drug, or a combination of drugs, you should complete this Yellow Card or complete a report on the website at www.yellowcard.gov.uk. For *intensively monitored medicines* (identified by ▼) report **all** suspected reactions (including any considered not to be serious). For *established drugs* and *herbal remedies* report **all serious** adverse reactions in adults; report **all serious and minor** adverse reactions in **children** (under 18 years). You do not have to be certain about causality: if in doubt, please report. Do not be put off reporting just because some details are not known. See BNF (page 11) or the MHRA website (www.yellowcard.gov.uk) for additional advice.

PATIENT DETAILS	Patient Initials:		Sex: M / F	Weight if known (kg):
Age (at time of reaction):		Identification (Your Practice / Hospital Ref.)*:		

SUSPECTED DRUG(S)

Give brand name of drug
and batch number if known

	Route	Dosage	Date started	Date stopped	Prescribed for

SUSPECTED REACTION(S)
Please describe the reaction(s) and any treatment given:

		Outcome
		Recovered ☐
		Recovering ☐
		Continuing ☐
		Other ☐

Date reaction(s) started: _____   Date reaction(s) stopped: _____

Do you consider the reaction to be serious?   Yes / No

If *yes*, please indicate why the reaction is considered to be serious (please tick all that apply):

Patient died due to reaction ☐	Involved or prolonged inpatient hospitalisation ☐
Life threatening ☐	Involved persistent or significant disability or incapacity ☐
Congenital abnormality ☐	Medically significant; please give details:

* This is to enable you to identify the patient in any future correspondence concerning this report

Please attach additional pages if necessary

Please list other drugs taken in the last 3 months prior to the reaction (including self-medication & herbal remedies)

Was the patient on any other medication?   Yes / No   If yes, please give the following information if known:

Drug (Brand, if known)	Route	Dosage	Date started	Date stopped	Prescribed for

Additional relevant information e.g. medical history, test results, known allergies, rechallenge (if performed), suspected drug interactions. For congenital abnormalities please state all other drugs taken during pregnancy and the date of the last menstrual period.

REPORTER DETAILS
Name and Professional Address:

Post code: _____   Tel No: _____

Speciality: _____

Signature: _____   Date: _____

CLINICIAN (if not the reporter)
Name and Professional Address:

Post code: _____

Tel No: _____   Speciality: _____

If you would like information about other adverse reactions associated with the suspected drug, please tick this box   ☐

If you report from an area served by a Yellow Card Centre (YCC), MHRA may ask the Centre to communicate with you, on its behalf, about your report. See BNF (page 11) for further details on YCCs. If you want only MHRA to contact you, please tick this box.   ☐

Send to **Medicines and Healthcare products Regulatory Agency, CHM FREEPOST, LONDON SW8 5BR**